THE NEW NON-ALCOHOLIC FATTY LIVER DISEASE DIET

Healthy Recipes for Reducing Liver Fat Accumulation, Detoxifying Your Body, and Improving Liver Functionality to Prevent Related Illnesses

Dr. Anna Fennell

COPYRIGHT

TABLE OF CONTENTS

DELICIOUS AND HEALTHY MAIN DISH RECIPES

INTRODUCTION

The escalating rates of obesity across the United States are starkly mirrored by the prevalence of non-alcoholic fatty liver disease (NAFLD), an ailment that arises when excess fat accumulates within liver cells, unrelated to alcohol consumption. This condition affects approximately one in every four individuals globally, signifying a considerable health burden on a worldwide scale.

When fatty tissue comprises more than 5% of the liver's total weight, NAFLD, colloquially termed as a "fatty liver," manifests. The deposition of excessive fat within the liver not only compromises its function but also poses an elevated risk for severe complications such as liver cancer or liver failure. Moreover, there exists a notable association between NAFLD and type 2 diabetes, with individuals affected by NAFLD being more prone to developing this metabolic disorder.

The confluence of obesity and other components of the metabolic syndrome serves as a primary driver for the prevalence of NAFLD. Projections indicate that by 2020, NAFLD is anticipated to emerge as the foremost cause of chronic liver disease, imposing a substantial economic burden, estimated at a staggering $292 billion annually in the United States alone.

NAFLD encompasses a spectrum of diseases, ranging from non-alcoholic fatty liver (NAFL) to the more severe non-alcoholic steatohepatitis (NASH), characterized by hepatic inflammation and cellular damage. NASH poses a significantly heightened risk of progressing to cirrhosis and hepatocellular carcinoma (HCC), making it a leading contributor to end-stage liver disease.

The hepatitis C virus (HCV) infection, once the predominant reason for liver transplantation in the United States, is now projected to be overtaken by NASH-related complications in the foreseeable future. This paradigm shift underscores the urgent need for effective interventions and management strategies to mitigate the escalating burden of NAFLD-related liver diseases.

Long-term follow-up studies among liver transplant recipients have identified NAFLD as a notable concern, emphasizing the importance of comprehensive care and monitoring post-transplantation. Moreover, the incidence of NAFLD-related HCC has witnessed a dramatic surge, driven by the burgeoning obesity epidemic, highlighting the imperative for concerted efforts in both prevention and treatment initiatives.

CHAPTER ONE

DEFINITION OF NON-ALCOHOLIC FATTY LIVER DISEASE (NAFLD)

Non-Alcoholic Fatty Liver Disease (NAFLD) is a condition characterized by the accumulation of fat in the liver cells (hepatocytes) of individuals who do not consume excessive alcohol. It is one of the most common liver disorders worldwide and is closely associated with obesity, insulin resistance, metabolic syndrome, and type 2 diabetes.

NAFLD encompasses a spectrum of liver conditions, ranging from simple steatosis (accumulation of fat) to non-alcoholic steatohepatitis (NASH), which involves inflammation and liver cell damage. In some cases, NAFLD can progress to more severe liver diseases such as fibrosis, cirrhosis, and even hepatocellular carcinoma (liver cancer).

The exact cause of NAFLD is not fully understood, but it is believed to be multifactorial, involving a combination of genetic, environmental, and lifestyle factors. Risk factors for NAFLD include obesity, insulin resistance, sedentary lifestyle, unhealthy diet (particularly high in sugar and saturated fats), and certain medical conditions such as metabolic syndrome and type 2 diabetes.

NAFLD is often asymptomatic in its early stages, and many individuals may remain unaware of their condition until it progresses to more advanced liver disease. However, some people with NAFLD may experience fatigue, abdominal discomfort, and an enlarged liver.

Diagnosis of NAFLD typically involves a combination of medical history assessment, physical examination, laboratory tests (including liver function tests and imaging studies such as ultrasound, CT scan, or MRI), and sometimes liver biopsy to assess the extent of liver damage.

Management of NAFLD focuses on lifestyle interventions aimed at reducing liver fat accumulation and preventing disease progression.

This includes dietary modifications to promote weight loss and improve insulin sensitivity, regular exercise, and treatment of underlying metabolic conditions such as diabetes and dyslipidemia. In more advanced cases, pharmacological therapies and bariatric surgery may be considered.

Early detection and management of NAFLD are crucial to preventing complications and improving long-term outcomes. Therefore, individuals at risk for NAFLD should undergo regular health screenings and adopt healthy lifestyle habits to protect liver health.

Causes and Risk Factors of NAFLD

Understanding these causes and risk factors is crucial for identifying individuals at risk of NAFLD and implementing preventive measures and early interventions to reduce the burden of the disease.

Causes:

1. Insulin Resistance: One of the primary underlying causes of NAFLD is insulin resistance, a condition in which the body's cells become less responsive to insulin. This leads to increased levels of insulin in the bloodstream, which can promote fat accumulation in the liver.

2. Metabolic Syndrome: NAFLD is closely associated with metabolic syndrome, a cluster of conditions including obesity, high blood pressure, abnormal lipid levels, and insulin resistance. These factors collectively contribute to the development and progression of fatty liver disease.

3. Genetics: Genetic factors play a role in predisposing individuals to NAFLD. Certain genetic variations can increase the likelihood of developing the disease, although lifestyle factors often interact with genetic predispositions.

4. Dietary Factors: Consumption of a diet high in calories, especially from sugars and unhealthy fats,

can contribute to the development of NAFLD. Excessive intake of refined carbohydrates, sugary beverages, and saturated fats can lead to increased fat deposition in the liver.

5. Sedentary Lifestyle: Lack of physical activity and a sedentary lifestyle are significant risk factors for NAFLD. Regular exercise helps improve insulin sensitivity, promotes weight loss, and reduces liver fat accumulation.

Risk Factors:

1. Obesity: Obesity, especially abdominal obesity (central adiposity), is strongly associated with

NAFLD. Excess body fat, particularly visceral fat surrounding abdominal organs, contributes to insulin resistance and fatty liver deposition.

2. Type 2 Diabetes: Individuals with type 2 diabetes are at higher risk of developing NAFLD due to insulin resistance and metabolic abnormalities. Conversely, NAFLD also increases the risk of developing type 2 diabetes, creating a bidirectional relationship between the two conditions.

3. High Cholesterol and Triglycerides: Elevated levels of cholesterol and triglycerides in the blood are associated with an increased risk of NAFLD. Dyslipidemia contributes to liver inflammation and the progression of fatty liver disease to more severe

forms such as non-alcoholic steatohepatitis (NASH).

4. Age and Gender: NAFLD can occur at any age but is more prevalent in middle-aged and older adults. Additionally, men tend to have a higher risk of NAFLD compared to premenopausal women, although the risk in women increases after menopause.

5. Ethnicity: Certain ethnic groups, such as Hispanic, South Asian, and Middle Eastern populations, have a higher prevalence of NAFLD compared to others. Genetic and lifestyle factors specific to these populations may contribute to increased susceptibility to the disease.

Types of NAFLD (Simple Fatty Liver vs. Non-Alcoholic Steatohepatitis - NASH)

1. Simple Fatty Liver (Steatosis):

 - In simple terms, this is the accumulation of fat in the liver without significant inflammation or liver cell damage.

 - It's considered the less severe form of NAFLD.

 - Individuals with simple fatty liver may not experience symptoms initially, and the condition may be discovered incidentally during medical tests for other reasons.

 - While it generally doesn't progress to serious liver disease in most cases, it can lead to non-alcoholic steatohepatitis (NASH) in some individuals.

- Management primarily focuses on lifestyle changes such as diet modification, regular exercise, and weight loss.

2. Non-Alcoholic Steatohepatitis (NASH):

- NASH is a more severe form of NAFLD characterized by liver inflammation and liver cell damage, in addition to fat accumulation in the liver.

- Unlike simple fatty liver, NASH can progress to more serious liver conditions such as cirrhosis, liver failure, and liver cancer.

- Symptoms may include fatigue, abdominal discomfort, enlarged liver, and elevated liver enzymes in blood tests.

- Diagnosis typically requires a liver biopsy to assess inflammation and liver damage.

- Management of NASH involves lifestyle changes (similar to simple fatty liver) but may also include medications aimed at reducing liver inflammation and fibrosis.

- It's important for individuals with NASH to be regularly monitored by healthcare providers to assess disease progression and to manage associated conditions such as diabetes and obesity effectively.

Understanding the differences between simple fatty liver and NASH is crucial for proper diagnosis, treatment, and management of NAFLD.

CHAPTER TWO

COMPREHENDING NON-ALCOHOLIC FATTY LIVER (NAFL)

The prevalence of non-alcoholic fatty liver disease (NAFLD) has surged in recent decades, encompassing a wider demographic than before. Estimates indicate its prevalence ranges from 24% to 32% in most industrialized nations, with developing nations experiencing rates around 25%. Notably, the Middle East exhibits the highest prevalence at 32%, contrasting with Africa's lower rate of 14%. In the United States alone, an estimated 83.1 million cases of NAFLD were recorded in 2015, with a prevalence rate of 25.8% across all age groups. However, it's noteworthy that only a minority, about 10%, of patients with severe fibrosis stemming from NAFLD progress to non-alcoholic steatohepatitis (NASH) during their clinical trajectory.

The existence of various disease risk factors distinctly influences NAFLD prevalence. Studies suggest incidence rates ranging from 30% to 100% among obese individuals, from 10% to 75% among those with Type 2 diabetes mellitus (T2DM), and from 20% to 92% among patients with hyperlipidemia. These prevalence variations are contingent upon factors such as age, ethnicity, and the presence of other comorbidities. Additionally, males exhibit a twofold higher likelihood of NAFLD compared to females, with prevalence increasing with age.

As the nomenclature implies, fatty liver disease denotes a medical condition characterized by the accumulation of fat in the liver. This condition manifests in two primary forms: alcohol-induced, attributable to excessive alcohol consumption, and non-alcoholic, which can occur even in individuals who abstain from alcohol consumption. While alcoholic fatty liver disease affects approximately 5% of the U.S. population, non-alcoholic fatty liver disease (NAFLD) impacts an estimated 100 million individuals in the United States alone, emerging as the most common liver disease even among children.

Non-alcoholic fatty liver steatohepatitis (NASH) represents a more severe manifestation of the disease, capable of progressing to dire conditions such as cirrhosis and liver cancer. Regardless of the subtype, lifestyle modification remains paramount in mitigating and potentially reversing the liver condition. This includes weight loss, abstaining from alcohol consumption, and adhering to a diet conducive to liver health.

The benefits of weight loss and an augmented protein intake in combatting NAFLD are noteworthy.

Recent studies have indicated promising findings suggesting that adopting a regimen focusing on weight loss and incorporating a high-protein diet may contribute significantly to reducing liver fat accumulation. In a meticulously conducted investigation involving 25 volunteers, researchers meticulously collected blood and urine samples, alongside conducting body scans, to meticulously evaluate the liver fat content and the elimination rate of proteins from the participants' bodies across three distinct intervals: six months later, followed by a subsequent assessment at the two-year mark, marking the initiation of the weight maintenance phase.

The results were intriguing; they revealed a notable correlation between the increase in protein consumption and diminished liver fat content after the sustained two-year period of weight management. Particularly noteworthy was the observation that over half of the participants previously diagnosed with non-alcoholic fatty liver disease (NAFLD) no longer exhibited indications of a fatty liver. This highlights the potential efficacy of a high-protein diet combined with sustained weight management in mitigating the progression of NAFLD and possibly even reversing its effects.

In addition to dietary modifications, maintaining a healthy weight is paramount in the prevention and management of NAFLD. Individuals who are overweight or obese should conscientiously monitor their daily calorie intake while simultaneously augmenting their physical activity levels. For those already within a healthy weight range, it is imperative to sustain these practices through continued adherence to a balanced diet and regular exercise routines.

Physical activity should be seamlessly integrated into one's daily routine to promote overall health and well-being. Even modest activities, such as a daily 30-minute walk, can serve as an auspicious starting point in fostering a more active lifestyle. By incorporating these lifestyle changes, individuals can proactively address the risk factors associated with NAFLD and promote liver health.

Symptoms of Non-Alcoholic Fatty Liver Disease

Non-Alcoholic Fatty Liver Disease (NAFLD) often manifests without obvious symptoms, making it a challenging condition to detect in its early stages. Symptoms, if present, tend to be nonspecific and can include fatigue and mild discomfort in the upper right abdomen. However, as the disease progresses, especially if it advances to cirrhosis, the symptoms may become more pronounced and diverse.

For individuals with advanced NAFLD or cirrhosis, symptoms may include male breast enlargement, the appearance of red palms, unexplained internal bruising, and fluid retention, which can lead to swelling in the abdomen and legs. These symptoms can significantly impact an individual's quality of life and may prompt further medical investigation.

To accurately diagnose NAFLD, a healthcare provider may recommend additional tests such as a fibroscan or liver biopsy. These diagnostic procedures help assess the extent of liver damage and determine the appropriate course of treatment.

While there is no specific medication to treat NAFLD, lifestyle modifications are key to managing the condition effectively. Gradual weight loss through a combination of a balanced diet and regular exercise is considered the cornerstone of treatment. Weight loss can help reduce the accumulation of fat in the liver, alleviate inflammation, and promote the healing of liver damage or scarring.

It's important for individuals diagnosed with NAFLD to work closely with their healthcare team to develop a personalized treatment plan tailored to their specific needs and health goals. Regular monitoring and follow-up appointments are essential to track progress, adjust treatment strategies as needed, and prevent potential complications associated with the disease.

CHAPTER THREE

DIAGNOSIS OF NON-ALCOHOLIC FATTY LIVER DISEASE

When individuals who are overweight or obese undergo routine blood tests and exhibit elevated liver values, healthcare providers often suspect the presence of fatty liver disease. Confirming the diagnosis of Non-Alcoholic Fatty Liver Disease (NAFLD) typically involves the utilization of imaging tests such as ultrasound or CT scans. These diagnostic tools enable doctors to visually inspect the liver for the accumulation of fat.

Moreover, advancements in medical technology now allow GCSA physicians to employ FibroScan technology to assess the level of scar tissue within the liver. This innovative approach facilitates a more comprehensive understanding of fatty liver disease, enabling healthcare professionals to categorize it into four distinct stages:

1. Steatosis/Fatty Liver: Characterized by the deposition of fat within liver cells.

2. Non-Alcoholic Steatohepatitis (NASH): Involves the presence of both scar tissue and liver inflammation.

3. Cirrhosis: A condition marked by the extensive replacement of liver cells with scar tissue, leading to significant impairment of liver function.

4. Liver Failure: Represents the endpoint of severe liver damage, where the liver is no longer able to carry out its vital functions, necessitating liver transplantation for survival.

This comprehensive classification system not only aids in diagnosing NAFLD but also provides valuable insights into disease progression and guides the implementation of appropriate treatment strategies tailored to each stage of the condition.

How can you ascertain whether you possess NAFLD?

Because non-alcoholic fatty liver disease often manifests without noticeable symptoms, it frequently remains undetected until incidental findings from routine tests or investigations for other health concerns uncover abnormalities in liver function. For instance, abnormalities may be observed on ultrasound imaging or through abnormal liver enzyme tests. In cases where initial tests yield inconclusive results or when there is a suspicion of liver disease, further diagnostic measures such as liver biopsy may be recommended by your healthcare provider. During a liver biopsy, a small sample of liver tissue is obtained using a needle inserted through the abdominal wall and into the liver. This tissue sample is then analyzed in a laboratory to assess for signs of inflammation, fibrosis, or other liver abnormalities, aiding in the diagnosis and management of non-alcoholic fatty liver disease and its potential progression to more severe conditions like non-alcoholic steatohepatitis (NASH) or cirrhosis. Thus, while NAFLD may not present obvious symptoms initially, timely diagnostic interventions such as liver biopsy can provide valuable insights into the state of liver health and guide appropriate treatment strategies.

Management and treatment of non-alcoholic fatty liver disease (NAFLD)

In the management of individuals across all risk categories who are diagnosed with NAFLD, lifestyle modifications emerge as a cornerstone. These modifications encompass abstaining from alcohol, shedding excess weight by aiming for a loss of 5-10% of body weight, and engaging in regular aerobic physical activities. The recommended physical activity regimen may include moderately intense sessions lasting between 150 to 300 minutes per week, vigorously intense sessions lasting between 75 to 150 minutes per week, or a combination of both. Furthermore, to achieve significant weight loss, a reduction in daily caloric intake by 500-1000 Kcal is advised.

Studies have shown that even a modest weight loss of more than 5% can lead to improvements in steatosis, while a weight loss exceeding 7% can result in the resolution of NASH. Additionally, a more substantial weight reduction exceeding 10% can induce regression in fibrosis. Beyond these direct effects on liver health, lifestyle changes leading to reduced liver fat and fibrosis in NAFLD patients have been linked to improved insulin sensitivity, a decreased risk of diabetes and cardiovascular diseases, and a lowered risk of progressive liver diseases, cirrhosis-related deaths, and hepatocellular carcinoma (HCC).

However, it's important to note potential challenges associated with weight loss efforts, such as the risk of muscle mass loss, exacerbation of sarcopenia, and nutrient deficiencies. Hence, seeking guidance from a nutrition specialist for a personalized care plan is advisable.

In cases where lifestyle modifications alone prove insufficient in achieving significant weight reduction, pharmacologic therapies utilizing FDA-approved agents for obesity may be warranted.

Regarding alcohol consumption, while there's limited clarity on the effects of light or moderate alcohol consumption in NAFLD patients, abstaining from alcohol is strongly advised, particularly in cases of advanced fibrosis.

On the other hand, moderate coffee consumption, typically defined as drinking 3-4 cups per day, has shown potential benefits in reducing gut permeability, improving fibrosis, and decreasing inflammation in NASH patients, thus it is highly recommended.

Pharmacologic interventions specifically aimed at resolving steatosis and fibrosis, and targeting factors involved in NASH pathogenesis, should also be considered. Statins and PPAR agonists, for instance, have demonstrated efficacy in reducing fat accumulation and metabolic features associated with NASH. Moreover, lifestyle modifications, medical interventions, endoscopic procedures, or surgical interventions that aid in weight reduction can complement the effects of these pharmacologic therapies.

Furthermore, the utilization of vitamins like Vitamin E has shown promise in NAFLD management, with studies demonstrating its ability to improve liver histology in non-diabetic individuals with biopsy-proven NASH.

Considering the potential side effects and contraindications, a comprehensive approach to treatment should be pursued, focusing on enhancing quality of life, preventing the progression of liver diseases, and mitigating systemic inflammation associated with metabolic syndrome.

Looking towards the future, numerous medications are currently under investigation in phase 2 and 3 clinical trials, either alone or in combination with weight loss interventions, which may hold promise in managing this severe epidemic of NAFLD.

Though it's premature to discuss their specifics at present, some noteworthy candidates include Cysteamine bitartrate, Cenicriviroc, Selonsertib, and Simtuzumab, among others.

CHAPTER FOUR

PREVENTING OF NON-ALCOHOLIC FATTY LIVER

Medical professionals often advise individuals on various steps to mitigate the likelihood of developing non-alcoholic fatty liver disease (NAFLD). One crucial recommendation involves adopting a nutritious diet that prioritizes certain food groups and limits others:

1. Embrace a Nutrient-Rich Diet: Opt for a diet abundant in fresh fruits, vegetables, whole grains,

and lean proteins. These foods provide essential vitamins, minerals, and antioxidants that support overall health and liver function.

2. Reduce Sugar Intake: High consumption of sugar, especially in the form of added sugars found in processed foods and sugary beverages, can contribute to liver fat accumulation. Minimizing intake of sugary snacks, desserts, and sweetened drinks helps lower the burden on the liver and reduces the risk of NAFLD development.

3. Limit Alcohol Consumption: Although NAFLD is not directly caused by alcohol consumption, excessive alcohol intake can exacerbate liver damage and increase the risk of liver-related complications. To safeguard liver health, it's

advisable to moderate alcohol consumption or avoid it altogether, especially for individuals with other risk factors for liver disease.

4. Practice Portion Control: Overeating and consuming large portion sizes can lead to weight gain and metabolic disturbances, both of which are risk factors for NAFLD. Monitoring portion sizes and practicing mindful eating can help maintain a healthy weight and reduce strain on the liver.

5. Stay Hydrated: Adequate hydration is essential for optimal liver function and overall health. Drinking plenty of water throughout the day supports liver detoxification processes and helps flush out toxins from the body.

By adhering to these dietary recommendations, individuals can proactively protect their liver health and reduce the likelihood of developing NAFLD. Additionally, incorporating regular physical activity, maintaining a healthy weight, and attending routine medical check-ups are integral components of a comprehensive approach to liver disease prevention.

8 foods to eat

Healthcare professionals often advise certain foods to promote a healthy liver. Here's a detailed exploration of some recommended dietary choices:

1. Almond Milk or Low-Fat Cow's Milk: Dr. Delgado-Borrego suggests almond milk or low-fat cow's milk for individuals, both adults and children, dealing with fatty liver disease. She emphasizes the potential benefits of adequate calcium and vitamin D intake in preventing the development of fatty liver disease. Moreover, patients with advanced liver disease often face multiple nutritional complications, including early osteopenia and osteoporosis. Despite the misconception that fatty liver disease reduces calcium absorption, Dr. Delgado-Borrego stresses that calcium is essential for everyone, recommending up to three glasses of either type of milk per day.

2. Coffee: Coffee, when consumed without added sugar or creamers, has emerged as a potential ally in combating fatty liver disease. Dr. Delgado-Borrego explains that coffee might reduce gut permeability, making it more challenging for people to absorb fats. While ongoing research is needed to fully understand this mechanism, mounting evidence suggests that coffee consumption can contribute to preventing fatty liver disease. Depending on the individual, multiple cups of coffee may be recommended.

3. Vitamin E-Rich Foods: Red bell peppers, spinach, peanuts, and nuts are rich sources of vitamin E, which can be beneficial for individuals with fatty liver. Further research is required, although initial

studies indicate modest improvements in individuals with non-alcoholic fatty liver disease (NAFLD) or non-alcoholic steatohepatitis (NASH) after consuming vitamin E-rich foods.

4. Water: It's essential to avoid sugary and calorie-dense beverages. Adequate water intake is crucial to prevent dehydration and its adverse effects on liver health. The general recommendation is to drink between half an ounce and an ounce of water for every pound of body weight per day, assuming no medical conditions that would restrict fluid intake.

5. Avocado Oil and Other Healthy Fats: Olive oil, avocado oil, and oils rich in monounsaturated fats, such as sesame, peanut, sunflower, canola, and safflower oil, are beneficial for liver health. These

oils help reduce liver enzyme levels and promote feelings of satiety. Additionally, plant-based sources of omega-3 fatty acids, such as flax and chia seeds, are recommended for their potential to decrease liver fat content.

6. Garlic: Increased intake of garlic, particularly through garlic powder, has shown promising results in reducing body fat mass and liver fat in patients with NAFLD. Incorporating garlic into the diet may help prevent the progression of fatty liver disease.

7. Soy Products: Some research suggests that soy products like tofu or soy milk may have a positive impact on fatty liver. Studies have indicated improvements in metabolic parameters in NAFLD patients following soy consumption.

These dietary recommendations, alongside lifestyle modifications and medical supervision, can play a significant role in managing and preventing fatty liver disease.

8 foods to stay away from

Typically, foods that can elevate blood sugar levels or contribute to weight gain are recommended to be avoided for individuals with concerns about their liver health. This advice is echoed by experts such as Dr. Delgado-Borrego, who emphasizes steering clear of beverages like juice, soda, and other sweetened drinks due to their high sugar and carbohydrate content, which can be detrimental to liver health.

Low-calorie diet beverages, often marketed as healthier alternatives, might not be the best choice according to Dr. Delgado-Borrego, as sugar substitutes in these drinks could potentially worsen liver disease.

Younan Brikho adds to this advice, cautioning against saturated fats commonly found in items like butter and ghee, which have been associated with increased triglyceride levels in the liver.

Moreover, sweet baked goods and desserts, including cakes, pastries, pies, ice cream, and similar treats, should be limited or avoided altogether for those aiming to address fatty liver disease due to their high sugar content.

Health specialists also discourage the consumption of bacon, sausage, cured meats, and fatty meats due to their high saturated fat content, which could exacerbate liver issues.

Furthermore, alcohol intake should be minimized or completely avoided, especially for individuals with fatty liver disease resulting from heavy drinking. While occasional alcohol consumption, such as a glass of wine, might be permissible for those with non-alcoholic fatty liver disease (NAFLD), it's essential to exercise caution.

Salt-heavy foods should also be limited, as research suggests that high salt consumption may worsen NAFLD by accompanying high-fat and high-calorie foods, potentially leading to further liver complications.

Additionally, fried foods, known for their calorie-dense nature, are advised against as they contradict the expert recommendation of following a more calorie-restricted diet, which is often beneficial for liver health.

In addition to dietary modifications, there are other lifestyle changes that can aid in reversing fatty liver disease:

1. Increasing physical activity: Regular exercise, as recommended by health experts, can significantly improve liver health. Dr. Delgado-Borrego suggests aiming for at least 60 minutes of physical activity daily, but this can be broken down into smaller increments for those finding it challenging.

2. Prioritizing sleep: Quality sleep is crucial, particularly for individuals with liver diseases. Conditions like obstructive sleep apnea can exacerbate liver issues, so ensuring adequate sleep duration and quality is essential.

3. Considering supplements: Before starting any supplements, it's advisable to consult a healthcare provider. Vitamin E, often used for liver problems, should be used cautiously to avoid adverse effects.

4. Exploring medication options: While there are currently no FDA-approved medications specifically for fatty liver disease, certain medications, such as pioglitazone, may be used off-label and have shown effectiveness in treating liver issues.

Ultimately, reversing fatty liver disease requires commitment to lifestyle changes, including dietary modifications, regular exercise, adequate sleep, and potentially supplementation or medication under medical supervision. The duration of recovery varies depending on individual factors such as weight loss progress and adherence to lifestyle changes. Additionally, reducing stress through lifestyle adjustments may also contribute to improving liver health, as cellular stress has been implicated in the development of fatty liver.

CHAPTER FIVE

DELICIOUS RECIPES FOR ELIMINATING NON-ALCOHOLIC FATTY LIVER DISEASE

DELICIOUS AND HEALTHY BREAKFAST RECIPES

Overnight Oatmeal with Milk

Things To Get

2 cups low-fat milk

2 cups rolled oats

1 teaspoon lemon zest

½ teaspoon vanilla extract

2 fresh apricots, chopped

⅓ cup pine nuts

2 tablespoons agave nectar (Optional)

Preparation

Combine milk, oats, lemon zest, and vanilla extract in a large bowl. Cover and refrigerate until oats have absorbed milk, 8 hours to overnight.

Stir apricots, pine nuts, and agave nectar into the oatmeal.

Note:

Use a milk substitute instead of the milk if preferred. Other seasonal fruit can be substituted for the apricots.

Diabetic-Friendly Apple Muffins

Things To Get

vegetable oil cooking spray

1 ⅔cups all-purpose flour

2 ½ teaspoons baking powder

1 tablespoon stevia sugar substitute

1 teaspoon ground cinnamon

½ teaspoon sea salt

¼ teaspoon nutmeg

⅔cup skim milk

1 egg, lightly beaten

¼ cup reduced-calorie margarine, melted

1 cup minced apple

Preparation

Preheat oven to 400 degrees F (200 degrees C). Prepare 12 muffin cups with cooking spray.

Mix flour, baking powder, stevia, cinnamon, sea salt, and nutmeg together in a large bowl. Beat skim milk, egg, and margarine together in a separate bowl; add to flour mixture and stir just until the dry mixture is moistened. Gently fold minced apple through the batter. Spoon batter into the prepared muffin cups.

Bake in preheated oven until lightly browned on the tops, about 25 minutes.

Daily Shake

Things To Get

½ cup Greek yogurt

½ cup almond milk

¼ cup fresh spinach

¼ cup fresh blueberries

1 tablespoon grapeseed oil

1 tablespoon ground chia seeds

1 tablespoon ground flax seed

1 tablespoon ground almonds

Preparation

Blend yogurt, almond milk, spinach, blueberries, grapeseed oil, chia seeds, flax seed, and almonds together in a blender until smooth.

Meyer Lemon Avocado Toast

Things To Get

2 slices whole grain bread

½ avocado

2 tablespoons chopped fresh cilantro, or more to taste

1 teaspoon Meyer lemon juice, or to taste

¼ teaspoon Meyer lemon zest

1 pinch cayenne pepper

1 pinch fine sea salt

¼ teaspoon chia seeds

Preparation

Toast bread slices to desired doneness, 3 to 5 minutes.

Mash avocado in a bowl; stir in cilantro, Meyer lemon juice, Meyer lemon zest, cayenne pepper, and sea salt. Spread avocado mixture onto toast and top with chia seeds.

Spinach Egg White Muffins

Things To Get

cooking spray

2 (4 ounce) cartons liquid egg whites

6 ounces shredded reduced-fat sharp Cheddar cheese, or more to taste

1 (10 ounce) package frozen chopped spinach, thawed and drained

1 teaspoon hot sauce

1 teaspoon salt

½ teaspoon ground black pepper

Preparation

Preheat the oven to 350 degrees F (175 degrees C). Spray a muffin tin with cooking spray.

Mix egg whites, Cheddar cheese, spinach, hot sauce, salt, and pepper in a bowl. Ladle mixture into the muffin tin, filling each cup 3/4 the way full.

Bake in the preheated oven until a knife inserted in the center of a muffin comes out clean, 20 to 25 minutes. Serve warm or cooled.

Overnight Light PB&J Oats

Things To Get

½ cup almond milk

¼ cup fresh raspberries

¼ cup rolled oats

2 tablespoons powdered peanut butter (such as PB2®)

1 ½ teaspoons chia seeds

1 teaspoon white sugar

Preparation

Mix almond milk, raspberries, rolled oats, powdered peanut butter, chia seeds, and sugar together in a container. Cover and refrigerate until oats are soft, 8 hours to overnight.

Spinach and Kale Smoothie

Things To Get

2 cups fresh spinach

1 cup almond milk

1 leaf kale

1 tablespoon peanut butter

1 tablespoon chia seeds (Optional)

1 sliced frozen banana

Preparation

Combine spinach, almond milk, kale, peanut butter, and chia seeds in a blender; blend until smooth. Add banana and blend until smooth.

Tips

You can substitute the spinach and kale with whatever greens you want.

Breakfast Egg Salad

Things To Get

1 tablespoon olive oil

¼ cup diced onion

1 rib celery, diced

¼ teaspoon dried rosemary

¼ teaspoon red pepper flakes (Optional)

salt and ground black pepper to taste

½ teaspoon minced garlic

1 egg

5 cherry tomatoes, quartered and seeded

1 tablespoon crumbled feta cheese, or more to taste

1 cup fresh spinach, torn into small pieces

Preparation

Heat oil in a large skillet over medium heat. Add onion, celery, rosemary, red pepper flakes, salt, and pepper; cook and stir with a wooden spoon or spatula until onion starts to turn translucent, about 4 minutes. Stir in garlic and cook for 1 minute.

Push onion mixture to outer edges of the skillet and crack egg into the middle. Break yolk with the wooden spoon and stir in onion mixture. Add tomatoes; cook and stir until egg is almost cooked, about 3 minutes. Stir in feta cheese until slightly melted, about 1 minute. Add spinach. Remove from heat and stir until slightly wilted, about 30 seconds.

Note: :

Substitute other leafy greens for the spinach if desired.

Dietetic Banana Nut Muffins

Things To Get

1 cup all-purpose flour

½ cup whole wheat flour

¾ cup granular sucrolose sweetener (such as Splenda®)

1 ¼ teaspoons baking powder

1 teaspoon baking soda

1 teaspoon ground cinnamon

2 egg whites

1 cup mashed ripe banana

¼ cup applesauce

Preparation

Preheat the oven to 375 degrees F (190 degrees C). Grease a 12 cup muffin tin, or line with paper muffin liners.

In a large bowl, stir together the flour, sugar substitute, baking powder, baking soda, and cinnamon. In a separate bowl, mix together the egg whites, mashed banana and applesauce. Add the wet **Things To Get**to the dry, and mix until just blended. Fill prepared muffin cups 3/4 full.

Bake for 15 to 18 minutes in the preheated oven, or until the top springs back when lightly touched. Allow muffins to cool in the pan over a wire rack for a little while before tapping them out of the pan.

Quinoa Breakfast Cereal

Things To Get

2 cups water

1 cup quinoa, rinsed

½ cup chopped dried apricots

½ cup slivered almonds

⅓ cup flax seeds

1 teaspoon ground cinnamon

½ teaspoon ground nutmeg

Preparation

Combine water and quinoa in a saucepan over medium heat; bring to a boil. Reduce heat and simmer until most of the water has been absorbed, 8 to 12 minutes. Stir in apricots, almonds, flax seeds, cinnamon, and nutmeg; cook until quinoa is tender, 2 to 3 minutes more.

Note:

If sweetness is desired, add a splash of maple syrup or honey.

Gluten-Free Hot Breakfast Cereal

Things To Get

1 cup brown basmati rice

½ cup quinoa

½ cup millet

½ cup buckwheat groats

½ cup sesame seeds

½ cup flax seeds

½ cup cornmeal

½ cup amaranth

Preparation

Grind the basmati rice in a coffee grinder until it resembles a coarse powder. Empty the ground rice into a bowl. Repeat the process with the quinoa, millet, buckwheat, sesame seeds, and flax seeds. Stir in the cornmeal and amaranth. Store in an air tight container in the refrigerator until ready to cook.

Foolproof Poached Eggs

Things To Get

4 organic eggs

2 teaspoons white vinegar

salt and ground black pepper to taste

1 pinch dried dill, or to taste

Preparation

Fill a large saucepan with 2 to 3 inches of water and bring to a simmer. Reduce the heat to medium-low, pour in vinegar, and keep the water at a gentle simmer.

Crack an egg into a small cup. Place cup near the surface of the hot water and gently drop egg into the water. Repeat with remaining eggs. Turn off heat, cover, and let sit until whites are set, 4 minutes. Lift eggs out of pan with a slotted spoon. Season with salt, pepper, and dill.

Note: :

I used organic eggs in this.

Healthy Multigrain Chia Waffles

Things To Get

cooking spray

1 ¾ cups almond milk

½ cup unsweetened applesauce

1 egg, beaten

2 tablespoons chia seeds

1 teaspoon vanilla extract

1 ¼ cups whole wheat flour

½ cup rolled oats

¼ cup flax seed meal

4 teaspoons baking powder

2 teaspoons white sugar, or more to taste

¼ teaspoon salt (Optional)

Preparation

Preheat a waffle iron according to the manufacturer's instructions; spray the inside with cooking spray.

Whisk almond milk, applesauce, egg, chia seeds, and vanilla extract together in a bowl; let sit until chia seeds start to thicken mixture, about 2 minutes.

Whisk flour, oats, flax seed meal, baking powder, sugar, and salt into almond milk mixture until batter is smooth.

Scoop 1/2 cup batter into the preheated waffle iron and cook until crisp and golden, about 5 minutes per waffle. Repeat with remaining batter.

Note:

These waffles freeze beautifully. Spray a baking sheet with cooking spray. Flash-freeze the waffles for 30 minutes. Place frozen waffles in a freezer bag. Toast individually frozen waffles in a toaster oven for 5 minutes. Before serving, place cooked waffles on paper towels to avoid sogginess.

Whole Grain French Toast with Blackberry Compote

Things To Get

2 (6 ounce) containers fresh blackberries

1 tablespoon honey (Optional)

1 egg, separated

1 egg white

¼ teaspoon ground nutmeg

¼ teaspoon ground cinnamon

¼ teaspoon ground ginger

5 slices whole-grain bread

Preparation

Place half the blackberries in a bowl; mash into a juicy pulp. Transfer to a small saucepan with the remaining blackberries. Cook over low heat until warm, 3 to 5 minutes. Add honey to the compote.

Beat egg yolk, egg whites, nutmeg, cinnamon, and ginger together in a bowl. Soak each slice of bread in the mixture for 10 to 15 seconds per side.

Heat a skillet over medium heat. Cook the soaked bread slices until golden brown, about 3 minutes per side. Ladle the warm berry compote on top.

Diabetic-Friendly Coconut Muffins

Things To Get

cooking spray

2 cups all-purpose flour

⅓ cup white sugar

¼ cup sweetened flaked coconut

2 teaspoons baking powder

¼ teaspoon salt

1 (8 ounce) container low-fat vanilla yogurt

1 large egg, lightly beaten

1 large egg white, lightly beaten

¼ cup vegetable oil

¼ teaspoon coconut extract

Preparation

Preheat oven to 400 degrees F (200 degrees C). Spray 12 muffin cups with cooking spray.

Stir flour, sugar, coconut, baking powder, and salt in a large bowl and make a well in the center. Whisk yogurt, egg, egg white, vegetable oil, and coconut extract together in a separate bowl until thoroughly combined. Pour egg mixture into well in dry **Things To Get**and stir just until moistened. Pour batter into prepared muffin cups, filling them 3/4 full.

Bake in the preheated oven until lightly browned, about 20 minutes. Remove muffins from pan immediately.

Avocado and Feta Egg White Omelet

Things To Get

½ cup egg whites

1 teaspoon paprika

½ tablespoon olive oil

3 leaves fresh basil

½ avocado, sliced

2 tablespoons crumbled feta cheese

Preparation

Mix egg whites and paprika together in a bowl.

Heat olive oil in a small skillet over medium heat.
Pour in egg white mixture; cook for 1 minute. Place

basil leaves over egg whites. Cook until egg white starts to firm up, about 1 minute. Spread avocado on top and sprinkle with feta cheese. Cook for 3 minutes more. Fold in half to form the omelet.

Healthy Wild Blueberry Sauce

Things To Get

3 cups frozen wild blueberries

⅓cup water

3 tablespoons honey

1 lemon, zested

1 pinch salt (Optional)

Preparation

Combine blueberries, water, honey, lemon zest, and salt in a saucepan over medium heat. Cover; bring to a simmer. Remove lid; simmer until liquids combine, about 15 minutes. Remove from heat; cool for 5 minutes.

Chia-Berry Swirl Oats

Things To Get

½ cup Quaker® Oats (Quick or Old Fashioned, uncooked)

1 cup water

½ cup fresh or frozen berries (blueberries, raspberries, and/or blackberries), thawed if frozen

1 tablespoon chia seeds

¼ teaspoon ground cinnamon

¼ teaspoon ground ginger

1 tablespoon plain nonfat yogurt, Greek or traditional

1 teaspoon unsweetened coconut

1 teaspoon honey

Preparation

In medium saucepan, bring water to a boil. Stir in oats. Cook uncovered over medium heat, 1 minute for Quick Oats, 5 minutes for Old Fashioned Oats, stirring occasionally.

Place berries, chia seeds, cinnamon, and ginger into blender or food processor container. Process until fruits are pureed. If mixture seems too thick, add water 1 tablespoon at a time to reach desired consistency. Swirl into bowl of cooked oats. Serve topped with yogurt, coconut, and honey.

Chia Greek Yogurt Pudding

Things To Get

1 cup unsweetened soy milk

1 cup Greek yogurt

2 tablespoons hulled hemp seeds

2 tablespoons ground flax seeds

1 tablespoon honey, or more to taste (Optional)

1 teaspoon ground cinnamon

1 teaspoon vanilla extract

⅔ cup chia seeds

Preparation

Whisk soy milk and Greek yogurt together in a large sealable container. Stir hemp seeds, flax seeds, honey, cinnamon, and vanilla extract into yogurt mixture.

Stir chia seeds into yogurt mixture until seeds are evenly distributed. Cover the container and refrigerate for 15 minutes. Stir mixture until chia seeds are evenly distributed again. Refrigerate until chilled and set, at least 1 hour.

DELICIOUS AND HEALTHY MAIN DISH RECIPES

Gnocchi

Things To Get

2 potatoes, peeled

2 cups all-purpose flour

1 egg

Preparation

Bring a large pot of salted water to a boil; add potatoes and cook until tender but still firm, about

15 minutes. Drain, cool, and mash with a fork or potato masher.

Combine 1 cup mashed potato, flour, and egg in a large bowl. Knead until dough forms a ball. Shape small portions of the dough into long "snakes". On a floured surface, cut snakes into 1/2-inch pieces.

Bring a large pot of lightly salted water to a boil. Drop in gnocchi and cook for 3 to 5 minutes or until gnocchi have risen to the top; drain and serve.

Black Beans and Rice

Things To Get

1 teaspoon olive oil

1 onion, chopped

2 cloves garlic, minced

¾ cup uncooked white rice

1 ½ cups low sodium, low fat vegetable broth

3 ½ cups canned black beans, drained

1 teaspoon ground cumin

¼ teaspoon cayenne pepper

Preparation

Heat oil in a saucepan over medium-high heat. Add onion and garlic; cook and stir until onion has softened, about 4 minutes. Stir in rice to coat; cook and stir for 2 minutes.

Add vegetable broth and bring to a boil. Cover, reduce to a simmer, and cook until liquid is absorbed, about 20 minutes.

Stir in beans, cumin, and cayenne; cook until beans are warmed through.

Slow Cooker Barbeque Chicken

Things To Get

4 skinless, boneless chicken breast halves

1 (18 ounce) bottle barbeque sauce (such as Sweet Baby Ray's®)

¼ cup distilled white vinegar

¼ cup brown sugar

1 teaspoon garlic powder

½ teaspoon red pepper flakes

Preparation

Place chicken breast halves in a slow cooker.

Whisk together barbeque sauce, vinegar, brown sugar, garlic powder, and pepper flakes in a bowl until sugar dissolves; pour over chicken.

Cook on Low for 4 to 6 hours.

Old Bay-Seasoned Steamed Shrimp

Things To Get

½ cup water

½ cup white vinegar

2 tablespoons seafood seasoning (such as Old Bay®)

1 pound fresh large shrimp, deveined with shells on

Preparation

Bring water, vinegar, and seafood seasoning to a boil in a saucepan over high heat. Add shrimp and stir.

Reduce heat to medium, cover, and steam, stirring once or twice, until bright orange in color, 3 to 5 minutes. Drain.

Slow Cooker Turkey Breast

Things To Get

1 (6 pound) bone-in turkey breast

1 (1 ounce) envelope dry onion soup mix

Preparation

Rinse turkey breast and pat dry. Cut off any excess skin, but leave the skin covering the breast. Rub onion soup mix all over outside of the turkey and under the skin.

Place in a slow cooker. Cover, and cook on High for 1 hour, then set to Low, and cook for 7 hours.

Red Lentil Curry

Things To Get

2 cups red lentils

3 cups water, or more as needed

1 tablespoon vegetable oil

1 large onion, diced

2 tablespoons curry paste

1 tablespoon curry powder

1 teaspoon ground turmeric

1 teaspoon ground cumin

1 teaspoon chili powder

1 teaspoon salt

1 teaspoon white sugar

1 teaspoon minced garlic

1 teaspoon minced fresh ginger

1 (14.25 ounce) can tomato puree

Preparation

Wash lentils in cold water until water runs clear.

Put lentils in a pot with enough water to cover;
bring to a boil and reduce heat to medium-low.
Cover and simmer, adding water as needed to keep
lentils covered, until tender, 15 to 20 minutes.
Drain.

Heat vegetable oil in a large skillet over medium heat; cook and stir onions in hot oil until caramelized, about 20 minutes.

Mix together curry paste, curry powder, turmeric, cumin, chili powder, salt, sugar, garlic, and ginger in a large bowl; stir into onions. Increase heat to high and cook, stirring constantly, until fragrant, 1 to 2 minutes.

Stir in tomato puree and lentils; cook until warmed through.

Fiesta Slow Cooker Shredded Chicken Tacos

Things To Get

1 cup chicken broth

3 tablespoons taco seasoning mix

1 pound skinless, boneless chicken breasts

Preparation

Combine chicken broth and taco seasoning mix in a bowl.

Place chicken in a slow cooker. Pour chicken broth mixture over chicken.

Cook on Low for 6 to 8 hours. Shred chicken.

Bourbon Chicken

Things To Get

4 skinless, boneless chicken breast halves

½ cup packed brown sugar

½ cup soy sauce

⅜ cup bourbon

2 tablespoons dried minced onion

1 teaspoon ground ginger

½ teaspoon garlic powder

Preparation

Place chicken breasts in a single layer in a 9x13-inch baking dish.

Mix together brown sugar, soy sauce, bourbon, dried minced onion, ginger, and garlic powder in a small bowl until well combined; pour over chicken. Cover the dish and marinate in the refrigerator for 8 hours to overnight.

Preheat the oven to 325 degrees F (165 degrees C).

Bake uncovered in the preheated oven, basting frequently, until chicken is well browned and juices run clear, about 1 1/2 hours. An instant-read thermometer inserted into the center should read at least 165 degrees F (74 degrees C).

Baked BBQ Chicken Tenders

Things To Get

cooking spray

⅓cup barbeque sauce (such as Sweet Baby Ray's® Hickory & Brown Sugar)

1 ½ tablespoons Asian-flavored barbeque seasoning (such as Savory Spice® Asian Delight BBQ Rub)

1 tablespoon caramel sauce

1 pound chicken tenders

Preparation

Preheat the oven to 375 degrees F (190 degrees C). Spray an 8x8-inch casserole dish with cooking spray.

Stir together barbeque sauce, barbeque seasoning, and caramel sauce in a shallow dish until combined. Reserve 2 tablespoons mixture for basting.

Dip each chicken tender into barbeque sauce mixture; coat thoroughly. Place in the prepared casserole dish.

Bake in the preheated oven until chicken is no longer pink in the center and the juices run clear, about 25 minutes. Baste with reserved sauce and bake 5 minutes more. An instant-read thermometer inserted into the center should read at least 165 degrees F (74 degrees C).

Vegan Black Bean Burgers

Things To Get

1 (15 ounce) can black beans, drained and rinsed

3 baby carrots, grated (Optional)

⅓cup chopped sweet onion

¼ cup minced green bell pepper (Optional)

1 tablespoon minced garlic

3 tablespoons chile-garlic sauce (such as Sriracha®), or to taste

1 tablespoon cornstarch

1 tablespoon warm water

1 teaspoon chili powder

1 teaspoon ground cumin

1 teaspoon seafood seasoning (such as Old Bay®)

¼ teaspoon salt

¼ teaspoon ground black pepper

2 slices whole-wheat bread, torn into small crumbs

¾ cup unbleached flour, or as needed

Preparation

Preheat the oven to 350 degrees F (175 degrees C). Grease a baking sheet.

Mash black beans in a bowl. Add carrots, onion, bell pepper, and garlic; mix well.

Whisk chile-garlic sauce, cornstarch, water, chili powder, cumin, seafood seasoning, salt, and black pepper together in a separate small bowl.

Stir chile-garlic sauce mixture into black bean mixture; mix in bread crumbs. Stir flour, 1/4 cup at a time, into bean mixture until a sticky batter forms.

Spoon mounds of batter onto the prepared baking sheet, about a 3/4-inch thickness per mound; shape into burgers.

Bake in the preheated oven until cooked in the center and crisp on the outside, about 10 minutes per side.

Tips

One egg can be substituted for cornstarch, but the recipe will not be vegan.

Porridge

Things To Get

2 ½ cups water

1 cup rolled oats

1 tablespoon white sugar

1 teaspoon salt

2 bananas, sliced

1 pinch ground cinnamon

½ cup cold milk (Optional)

Preparation

Combine water, oats, sugar, and salt in a saucepan. Add bananas and cinnamon. Bring to a boil, then reduce heat to low, and simmer until the liquid has been absorbed, stirring frequently.

Pour into bowls, and top each with a splash of cold milk.

Steamed Blue Crabs

Things To Get

3 cups beer

3 cups distilled white vinegar

¾ cup seafood seasoning (such as Old Bay®), divided

½ cup salt

36 live blue crabs

Preparation

Combine beer, vinegar, 1/2 cup seafood seasoning, and salt in a large stockpot over high heat. Bring to a strong simmer.

Right before cooking, carefully place each crab upside down and stick a knife through the shell, just behind the mouth.

Fit a screen over simmering beer mixture and layer crabs on the screen.

Cover and steam crabs until they turn bright orange and no blue-green color remains, 20 to 30 minutes. Sprinkle with remaining 1/4 cup seafood seasoning before serving.

Note:

The nutrition data for this recipe includes the full amount of salt used in the boiling liquid. The actual amount of salt consumed will vary.

Eggless Pasta

Things To Get

2 cups semolina flour

½ teaspoon salt

½ cup warm water, or more as needed

Preparation

Mix flour and salt together in a large bowl. Add warm water and stir to make a stiff dough; add more water if dough seems too dry.

Pat dough into a ball and turn out onto a lightly floured surface. Knead for 10 to 15 minutes. Cover and let rest for 20 minutes.

Working with 1/4 of the dough at a time and keeping the rest covered to prevent it from drying out, roll dough by hand to a thickness of 1/16 inch. If using a pasta machine, stop at the third to the last setting. Cut pasta into desired shapes.

Bring a large pot of lightly salted water to a boil. Cook pasta in the boiling water until tender yet firm to the bite, 3 to 5 minutes. Drain.

Homemade Puréed Sweet Potato Baby Food

Things To Get

2 sweet potatoes, peeled and halved, or more as desired

water to cover

Preparation

Fill a small saucepan with water; add sweet potatoes. Bring water to a boil and cook sweet potatoes until tender enough to break apart with a fork, 25 to 30 minutes.

Transfer sweet potatoes to a food processor or an immersion blender cup, reserving the cooking water. Blend sweet potatoes until smooth. Add 1/2 to 3/4 cup cooking water and blend until desired consistency is reached.

Tips

Breast milk or formula can be used instead of cooking water. Please consult your pediatrician before starting your baby on solid foods.

Egg Fried Rice

Things To Get

1 cup water

2 tablespoons soy sauce

½ teaspoon salt

1 cup uncooked instant rice

1 teaspoon vegetable oil

½ onion, finely chopped

½ cup green beans

1 large egg, lightly beaten

¼ teaspoon ground black pepper

Preparation

Bring water, soy sauce, and salt to a boil in a medium saucepan. Stir in rice and remove from heat. Cover and let stand for 5 minutes.

Heat oil in a medium skillet or wok over medium heat. Sauté onions and green beans in hot oil for 2 to 3 minutes. Pour in beaten egg and fry for 2 minutes, scrambling egg while it cooks.

Add cooked rice to egg mixture; mix well. Season with pepper.

Chicken Satay

Things To Get

2 tablespoons creamy peanut butter

½ cup soy sauce

½ cup lemon or lime juice

1 tablespoon brown sugar

2 tablespoons curry powder

2 cloves garlic, chopped

1 teaspoon hot pepper sauce

6 skinless, boneless chicken breast halves - cubed

Preparation

In a mixing bowl, combine peanut butter, soy sauce, lime juice, brown sugar, curry powder, garlic and hot pepper sauce. Place the chicken breasts in the marinade and refrigerate. Let the chicken marinate at least 2 hours, overnight is best.

Preheat a grill to high heat.

Weave the chicken onto skewers, then grill for 5 minutes per side.

Easy Garlic and Rosemary Chicken

Things To Get

2 skinless, boneless chicken breasts

2 cloves garlic, chopped

2 tablespoons dried rosemary

1 tablespoon lemon juice

salt and pepper to taste

Preparation

Preheat the oven to 375 degrees F (190 degrees C).

Cover chicken breasts with garlic, then sprinkle with rosemary, lemon juice, and salt and pepper to taste.

Place in a 9x13-inch baking dish and bake in the preheated oven until done and juices run clear, about 25 minutes (baking time will depend on the thickness of your chicken breasts).

French Toast Sticks

Things To Get

2 large eggs

½ cup powdered sugar

¼ cup milk

2 tablespoons maple syrup

1 teaspoon brown sugar

¼ teaspoon ground cinnamon

6 slices white bread, cut into thirds

nonstick cooking spray

Preparation

Mix eggs, powdered sugar, milk, maple syrup, brown sugar, and cinnamon together in a bowl with a fork until well blended. Dip each bread stick into the egg mixture.

Coat a skillet with nonstick spray and heat over medium heat. Place sticks in the hot skillet and cook until brown, 2 to 3 minutes; turn over and cook until browned on other side, 2 to 3 minutes more. Repeat with the second batch.

Note: :

Sticks can be frozen. Let them cool and then wrap desired amount in waxed paper and place in a freezer bag. To reheat, take out a small package and heat in a microwave for 1 minute to 1 minute 15 seconds, depending on how many.

Pierogi Dough

Things To Get

4 cups all-purpose flour

1 teaspoon salt

2 teaspoons vegetable oil

¼ teaspoon baking powder

1 cup warm water

1 egg, beaten

Preparation

In a large bowl mix together the flour, salt, and baking powder. Make a well in the center.

In a separate bowl mix together the vegetable oil, warm water, and beaten egg. Pour into the well of the dry Ingredients. Knead dough for 8 to 10 minutes.

Cover dough and let rest for 2 hours. Roll out and fill as desired.

Potato Dumplings

Things To Get

2 large potatoes, peeled and chopped

1 cup self-rising flour

1 egg

8 large seasoned croutons

Preparation

Bring a large pot of salted water to a boil. Add potatoes and cook until tender, about 15 minutes. Drain and mash.

In a medium bowl combine 2 cups mashed potatoes with flour and egg. Using about 1/4 to 1/2 cup of mixture each, shape into dumplings. Press a crouton into the center of each and seal dough around it.

Drop dumplings into simmering soup or broth, cover and cook 20 minutes. Do not remove lid while dumplings are cooking.

Pioneer Cut Dumplings from the 1800's

Things To Get

3 cups all-purpose flour

1 ½ teaspoons salt

1 egg

1 cup milk

Preparation

In a medium bowl, stir together the flour and salt. Add the milk and egg, and mix until it forms a dough. Knead on a lightly floured surface until smooth. Roll out to your desired thickness for dumplings or you can roll thinner for noodles. Cut into strips, squares, or any shape you like. Let dry while you prepare broth or soup.

Drop dumplings into boiling broth, and cook until tender. Time will depend on the thickness of the dumplings and how dry they were.

Homemade Gluten-Free Gnocchi

Things To Get

1 ½ pounds potatoes

1 egg at room temperature, lightly beaten

⅓ cup potato starch

1 tablespoon sweet rice flour

½ teaspoon fine salt

2 tablespoons rice flour, or as needed

Preparation

Preheat the oven to 400 degrees F (200 degrees C). Prick each potato a few times with a fork and place on a baking sheet.

Bake potatoes in the preheated oven until tender when pierced with a knife, about 50 minutes. Cool until easily handled, about 10 minutes.

Peel potatoes and pass through a ricer or food mill into a large bowl. Make a well in the center and pour in egg; mix well.

Whisk potato starch, sweet rice flour, and salt together in a bowl. Sprinkle over potato mixture; stir until a soft dough has formed. Cut dough into 4 equal parts with a knife or pastry cutter.

Dust the work surface with rice flour to keep dough from sticking. Roll out 1 piece of dough into a rope about 1 inch in diameter. Cut into 1-inch gnocchi.

Gently roll each one with the back of a fork to create ridges. Repeat with remaining dough.

Shake off any excess rice flour and let gnocchi rest, about 5 minutes.

Bring a large pot of salted water to a boil. Add gnocchi in batches and cook, without stirring, until they float to the top, 1 to 2 minutes. Remove with a slotted spoon.

Tips

Substitute arrowroot flour for the sweet rice flour if desired. If not cooking right away, roll the gnocchi in rice flour and arrange on a baking sheet about 1/4 inch apart. Let rest, about 5 minutes. Refrigerate for up to 24 hours or freeze up to 6 months. (Once cooled or frozen, the gnocchi won't stick together so you can transfer them from the baking sheet to freezer bags.) Frozen gnocchi will take about 3 minutes to cook. Thawed, they can be added directly to your favorite sauce that has already been heated. The texture of cooled or frozen gnocchi may differ from fresh.

Lemony Steamed Fish

Things To Get

6 (6 ounce) halibut fillets

1 tablespoon dried dill weed

1 tablespoon onion powder

2 teaspoons dried parsley

¼ teaspoon paprika

1 pinch seasoned salt, or more to taste

1 pinch lemon pepper

1 pinch garlic powder

2 tablespoons lemon juice

Preparation

Preheat oven to 375 degrees F (190 degrees C).

Cut 6 foil squares large enough for each fillet.

Center fillets on the foil squares and sprinkle each with dill weed, onion powder, parsley, paprika, seasoned salt, lemon pepper, and garlic powder. Sprinkle lemon juice over each fillet. Fold foil over fillets to make a pocket and fold the edges to seal. Place sealed packets on a baking sheet.

Bake in the preheated oven until fish flakes easily with a fork, about 30 minutes.

Air Fryer Fresh-Caught Crappie

Things To Get

1 pound fresh crappie fillets

2 tablespoons salt

½ cup yellow cornmeal

¼ cup all-purpose flour

1 teaspoon seasoned salt (such as LAWRY'S®)

1 teaspoon paprika

½ teaspoon ground black pepper

¼ teaspoon cayenne pepper (Optional)

cooking spray

Preparation

Place crappie fillets in a bowl. Add salt and water to cover. Cover and let sit to draw out all the blood, about 30 minutes. Rinse fillets thoroughly to remove salt. Pat dry with paper towels.

Preheat the air fryer to 400 degrees F (200 degrees C) according to manufacturer's instructions.

Add cornmeal, flour, seasoned salt, paprika, pepper, and cayenne to a gallon-sized zip-top bag. Seal and shake until evenly combined. Drop 2 fillets into the bag, seal, and shake to coat. Transfer to a plate. Repeat with remaining fillets.

Spray the tops of the fillets with nonstick cooking spray. Place a layer of fillets in the air fryer basket, sprayed-side down, making sure none are overlapping. Spray the tops with cooking spray. Cook for 4 minutes. Carefully flip and spray any chalky spots. Cook until crispy, about 4 minutes more. Repeat with remaining fillets.

Note:

Nutrition data for this recipe includes the full amount of brining Ingredients. The actual amount of brine consumed will vary.

Japanese Pan Noodles

Things To Get

1 (10 ounce) package fresh udon noodles

½ teaspoon sesame oil, divided, or to taste

2 cups chopped broccoli

½ green bell pepper, cut into matchsticks

2 small carrots, cut into matchsticks, or to taste

½ zucchini, thinly sliced

2 tablespoons soy sauce

2 tablespoons mirin (Japanese sweet wine)

1 tablespoon chili-garlic sauce

¾ teaspoon minced ginger

Preparation

Bring a large pot of lightly salted water to a boil. Cook udon in boiling water, stirring occasionally, until noodles are tender yet firm to the bite, 10 to 12 minutes. Drain and rinse with cold water. Stir in a few drops of sesame oil.

Heat the remaining sesame oil in a large skillet over medium heat. Cook broccoli until bright green and still crunchy, about 5 minutes. Add green bell pepper and carrots; cook and stir until slightly softened, about 2 minutes. Add zucchini; cook until slightly softened, about 2 minutes more. Add soy sauce, mirin, chili-garlic sauce, and ginger; stir to combine. Mix in the noodles; cook and stir until noodles absorb some of the sauce, 1 to 2 minutes more.

Note:

You can use any vegetables you want. I like to add bamboo shoots, bok choy, onion, etc. You can add any kind of protein.

Slow Cooker Salsa Chicken

Things To Get

2 pounds skinless, boneless chicken

2 tablespoons taco seasoning mix

1 cup diced tomatoes with habaneros (such as RO*TEL® Hot)

1 cup finely chopped onion

½ cup finely chopped celery

½ cup shredded carrot

1 cup prepared salsa

¼ cup water

Preparation

Put chicken into the crock of a slow cooker. Sprinkle taco seasoning over the chicken. Layer diced tomatoes with habaneros, onion, celery, and carrot over the chicken, respectively; top with salsa. Pour water over the entire mixture.

Cook on Low until the chicken is easily shreddable, 6 to 8 hours. An instant-read thermometer should read 165 degrees F (74 degrees C).

Shred the chicken with 2 forks and stir with the salsa mixture.

Note:

As a low-carb option just serve in a bowl, similar to stew, and top with grated cheese, sour cream, cilantro, and chopped scallions.

Great for filling tacos and burritos or even as the meat for a tortilla soup. Use your imagination to create other menu ideas.

Sweet Potato Gnocchi

Things To Get

2 (8 ounce) sweet potatoes

1 clove garlic, pressed

½ teaspoon salt

½ teaspoon ground nutmeg

1 egg

2 cups all-purpose flour

Preparation

Preheat the oven to 350 degrees F (175 degrees C). Bake sweet potatoes for 30 minutes, or until soft to the touch. Remove from the oven, and set aside to cool.

Once the potatoes are cool enough to work with, remove the peels, and mash them, or press them through a ricer into a large bowl. Blend in the garlic, salt, nutmeg, and egg. Mix in the flour a little at a time until you have soft dough. Use more or less flour as needed.

Bring a large pot of lightly salted water to a boil. While you wait for the water, make the gnocchi. On a floured surface, roll the dough out in several long snakes, and cut into 1-inch sections. Drop the pieces into the boiling water, and allow them to cook until they float to the surface. Remove the floating pieces with a slotted spoon, and keep warm in a serving dish. Serve with butter or cream sauce.

Easy Homemade Dumplings

Things To Get

2 cups all-purpose flour

2 teaspoons baking powder

1 teaspoon salt

1 cup milk

Preparation

Whisk flour, baking powder, and salt together in a bowl. Slowly pour milk into flour mixture, stirring constantly until dough is stiff and holds together.

Note:

Drop 1 tablespoon dough into the simmering stew or broth. Cook until dumpling is cooked through and fluffy, about 10 minutes per side.

Super Easy Slow Cooker Chicken Enchilada Meat

Things To Get

2 cups chicken broth

1 (14.5 ounce) can diced tomatoes

⅓cup chili powder

½ cup all-purpose flour

1 clove garlic

2 teaspoons ground cumin

1 teaspoon oregano

1 teaspoon salt, or to taste

1 pinch cayenne pepper, or more to taste (Optional)

4 skinless, boneless chicken breast halves

Preparation

Blend chicken broth, tomatoes, chili powder, flour, garlic, cumin, oregano, salt, and cayenne pepper in a blender until smooth.

Put chicken breast in bottom of a slow cooker; pour blended enchilada sauce over the chicken.

Cook on Low 8 to 9 hours (or 4 to 6 hours on High). Shred the chicken with 2 large forks and stir into the sauce.

Slow Cooker Boneless Turkey Breast

Things To Get

1 (10 pound) boneless turkey breast

2 (1 ounce) packages dry onion soup mix

¾ cup water

2 tablespoons garlic powder

2 tablespoons onion powder

1 tablespoon dried parsley

1 tablespoon seasoned salt (such as Season-All®)

1 tablespoon dried basil

1 tablespoon dried oregano

Preparation

Place turkey breast into a large slow cooker. Whisk onion soup mix and water in a bowl and pour the mixture over the turkey breast, spreading it out to evenly cover the meat.

Stir garlic powder, onion powder, parsley, seasoned salt, basil, and oregano in a bowl until thoroughly combined; sprinkle the seasonings over the turkey breast.

Cook on Low until turkey is very tender and the seasonings have flavored the meat, 8 to 9 hours. An instant-read meat thermometer inserted into the thickest part of the breast should read at least 165 degrees F (75 degrees C).

Instant Pot Apple Pie Steel Cut Oats

Things To Get

3 cups water

1 cup steel-cut oats

1 apple, or more to taste, chopped

1 ½ teaspoons ground cinnamon

½ teaspoon salt

¼ teaspoon ground nutmeg

Preparation

Combine water, oats, apple, cinnamon, salt, and nutmeg in a multi-functional pressure cooker (such as Instant Pot®). Close and lock the lid. Seal vent. Select Manual function; set timer for 5 minutes. Allow 10 to 15 minutes for pressure to build.

Release pressure using the natural-release method according to manufacturer's instructions, about 10 minutes. Release remaining pressure naturally. Stir and remove pot carefully with oven mitts.

Orange, Honey and Soy Chicken

Things To Get

2 skinless, boneless chicken breast halves, diced

2 oranges, juiced

¼ cup soy sauce

¼ cup honey

1 tablespoon garlic paste

1 tablespoon ginger paste

ground black pepper to taste

Preparation

Combine chicken, orange juice, soy sauce, honey, garlic paste, ginger paste, and black pepper in a large nonstick skillet over medium-high heat. Cook and stir until the sauce reduces to a sticky glaze and the chicken is cooked through, about 20 minutes.

Portuguese Shrimp

Things To Get

1 tablespoon extra-virgin olive oil, or more as needed

1 onion, chopped

3 cloves garlic, minced

1 (12 fluid ounce) can ale, divided

5 sprigs parsley, stemmed and chopped

2 teaspoons tomato paste

2 teaspoons Portuguese hot pepper sauce (pimenta)

1 cube chicken bouillon

1 teaspoon ground paprika

2 pounds unpeeled large shrimp, deveined

1 teaspoon kosher salt

Preparation

Heat olive oil in a large skillet over medium heat. Add onion and garlic; cook and stir until softened, about 5 minutes. Stir in parsley, tomato paste, hot pepper sauce, chicken bouillon, and paprika. Pour in half of the ale; simmer until flavors combine, about 5 minutes.

Pour remaining ale into the skillet; add shrimp. Season with salt. Cook until shrimp absorbs the liquid and turns pink, 15 to 20 minutes.

Instant Pot Shredded Chicken

Things To Get

4 pounds skinless, boneless chicken breasts

½ cup water

1 teaspoon salt

½ teaspoon ground black pepper

Preparation

Combine chicken breasts, water, salt, and pepper in a multi-functional pressure cooker (such as Instant Pot®). Close and lock the lid. Select high pressure according to manufacturer's instructions; set timer for 20 minutes. Allow 10 to 15 minutes for pressure to build.

Release pressure carefully using the quick-release method according to manufacturer's instructions, about 5 minutes. Unlock and remove the lid.

Shred the chicken using 2 forks. Store shredded chicken in an airtight container with the liquid to help keep it moist.

Note:

Substitute chicken broth for the water if preferred.

Quinoa Porridge

Things To Get

½ cup quinoa

¼ teaspoon ground cinnamon

1 ½ cups almond milk

½ cup water

2 tablespoons brown sugar

1 teaspoon vanilla extract (Optional)

1 pinch salt

Preparation

Heat a saucepan over medium heat and measure in
the quinoa. Season with cinnamon and cook until

toasted, stirring frequently, about 3 minutes. Pour in the almond milk, water and vanilla and stir in the brown sugar and salt. Bring to a boil, then cook over low heat until the porridge is thick and grains are tender, about 25 minutes. Add more water if needed if the liquid has dried up before it finishes cooking. Stir occasionally, especially at the end, to prevent burning.

Corned Venison

Things To Get

2 cups water

6 tablespoons sugar-based curing mixture (such as Morton® Tender Quick®)

½ cup brown sugar

4 ½ teaspoons pickling spice

1 tablespoon garlic powder

6 cups cold water

5 pounds boneless shoulder venison roast

Preparation

Bring 2 cups of water to a boil in a saucepan over high heat. Stir in the curing mixture, brown sugar, pickling spice, and garlic powder; stir until dissolved then remove from the heat. Pour 6 cups of cold water into a 2-gallon container, and stir in the spice mixture. Place the boneless venison into the brine, cover and refrigerate.

Leave the venison in the refrigerator to brine for 5 days, turning the meat over every day.

To cook, rinse the meat well, place into a large pot, and cover with water. Bring to a boil, then reduce heat to medium-low, cover, and simmer for 4 hours. Remove the venison from the pot, and allow to rest for 30 minutes before slicing.

Note:

You may freeze uncooked corned venison by placing the desired amounts in vacuum sealable bags. Do not rinse meat before freezing, but remove excess liquid before sealing.

Hawaiian Pork Hash

Things To Get

¼ pound ground pork

¼ pound shrimp - peeled, deveined and minced to a paste

1 egg white

2 tablespoons chopped water chestnuts

2 tablespoons chopped green onion

2 tablespoons cornstarch

2 teaspoons soy sauce

1 teaspoon white sugar

1 teaspoon minced garlic

1 teaspoon oyster sauce

¼ teaspoon salt

¼ teaspoon ground black pepper

¼ teaspoon sesame oil

1 (14 ounce) package round dumpling skins

Preparation

In a medium bowl, mix together the ground pork, shrimp, egg white, water chestnuts, green onion, cornstarch, soy sauce, sugar, garlic, oyster sauce, salt, pepper, and sesame oil.

Place about 1 tablespoon of this filling onto the center of each dumpling wrapper, and bring the sides up to the top. Do not seal the top, as these dumplings are left open. Place dumplings in a steamer.

Set the steamer basket over a pan or wok of boiling water. Steam for 30 minutes.

Reduced Fat French Toast

Things To Get

½ cup egg substitute

⅔cup skim milk

1 teaspoon vanilla extract

½ teaspoon ground cinnamon

6 slices reduced calorie white bread

Preparation

Beat together egg substitute, milk, vanilla and cinnamon. Dip bread slices in egg mixture until both sides are soaked.

Spray a skillet or frying pan with cooking spray and heat over medium high heat. Place bread slices into pan and cook until golden brown on both sides

Meyer Lemon Avocado Toast

Things To Get

2 slices whole grain bread

½ avocado

2 tablespoons chopped fresh cilantro, or more to taste

1 teaspoon Meyer lemon juice, or to taste

¼ teaspoon Meyer lemon zest

1 pinch cayenne pepper

1 pinch fine sea salt

¼ teaspoon chia seeds

Preparation

Toast bread slices to desired doneness, 3 to 5 minutes.

Mash avocado in a bowl; stir in cilantro, Meyer lemon juice, Meyer lemon zest, cayenne pepper, and sea salt. Spread avocado mixture onto toast and top with chia seeds.

Cinnamon Chicken

Things To Get

4 skinless, boneless chicken breast halves

1 teaspoon ground cinnamon

2 tablespoons Italian-style seasoning

1 ½ teaspoons garlic powder

3 teaspoons salt

1 teaspoon ground black pepper

Preparation

Preheat oven to 350 degrees F (175 degrees C).

Place chicken in a lightly greased 9x13 inch baking dish. Sprinkle evenly with ground cinnamon, seasoning, garlic powder, salt and pepper. (Note: You can be liberal with the seasoning, garlic powder, salt and pepper; however, the cinnamon should only be a dusting and not clumped.)

Bake at 350 degrees F (175 degrees C) for about 30 minutes or until chicken is cooked through and juices run clear.

Jenny's Grilled Chicken Breasts

Things To Get

4 skinless, boneless chicken breast halves

½ cup lemon juice

½ teaspoon onion powder

ground black pepper to taste

seasoning salt to taste

2 teaspoons dried parsley

Preparation

Preheat an outdoor grill for medium-high heat, and lightly oil grate.

Dip chicken in lemon juice, and sprinkle with the onion powder, ground black pepper, seasoning salt and parsley. Discard any remaining lemon juice.

Cook on the prepared grill 10 to 15 minutes per side, or until no longer pink and juices run clear.

Spaghetti With Marinara Sauce

Things To Get

1 pound spaghetti

1 (28 ounce) can crushed tomatoes

1 (14.5 ounce) can diced tomatoes

1 (15 ounce) can tomato sauce

1 tablespoon minced garlic

2 teaspoons white sugar

2 teaspoons dried parsley

1 teaspoon garlic powder

½ teaspoon salt

¼ teaspoon dried oregano

¼ teaspoon dried basil

¼ teaspoon ground black pepper

1 ½ tablespoons capers

1 pinch crushed red pepper flakes (Optional)

Preparation

In a large saucepan combine crushed tomatoes, diced tomatoes, tomato sauce, minced garlic, sugar, parsley, garlic powder, salt, oregano, basil, and ground black pepper. Add capers and crushed red pepper if desired. Cover. Bring to a boil.

Lower heat and simmer, with cover, for 45 to 60 minutes.

As simmering time nears, in a large pot with boiling salted water cook spaghetti until al dente.

Toss spaghetti with cooked sauce. Serve warm.

Easy BBQ Bake

Things To Get

¾ cup barbecue sauce

¾ cup honey

½ cup ketchup

1 onion, chopped

4 skinless, boneless chicken breast halves

Preparation

Preheat oven to 400 degrees F (200 degrees C).

In a medium bowl, combine the barbecue sauce, honey, ketchup and onion and mix well. Place chicken in a 9x13 inch baking dish. Pour sauce over the chicken and cover dish with foil.

Bake at 400 degrees F (200 degrees C) for 45 minutes to 1 hour, or until chicken juices run clear.

Chicken Diane Style

Things To Get

2 small onions, chopped

1 pound fresh mushrooms

8 skinless, boneless chicken breast halves

½ teaspoon salt

½ teaspoon ground black pepper

½ teaspoon paprika

2 teaspoons chopped fresh chives

2 teaspoons dried parsley

½ cup chicken broth

¼ cup brandy

2 tablespoons prepared Dijon-style mustard

Preparation

Saute onions and mushrooms in a large skillet over medium heat. Remove onion/mushroom mixture from skillet and reserve; add chicken breasts to skillet. Saute for 4 minutes, then turn over and add mushroom mixture on top.

In a small bowl mix salt, pepper, paprika, chives and parsley together then sprinkle mixture over chicken. In a medium bowl combine the broth, brandy and mustard and blend together. Pour over chicken, reduce heat to low and simmer for 20 to 25 minutes or until chicken is cooked through (no longer pink inside).

Low-Cal Chicken

Things To Get

4 (4 ounce) skinless, boneless chicken breast halves

1 ½ tablespoons minced onion

2 tablespoons crushed garlic

1 ½ teaspoons poultry seasoning

¼ cup soy sauce

2 teaspoons artificial sweetener

Preparation

Preheat oven to 425 degrees F (220 degrees C).

Place chicken in a 9x13 inch baking dish; sprinkle with onion, garlic, seasoning, soy sauce and sweetener.

Place foil over pan and bake for one hour at 425 degrees F (220 degrees C). It's ready to serve!

Honey Soy Tilapia

Things To Get

3 tablespoons honey

3 tablespoons soy sauce

3 tablespoons balsamic vinegar

1 tablespoon minced garlic

2 (3 ounce) fillets tilapia

cooking spray

1 teaspoon freshly cracked black pepper

Preparation

Mix the honey, soy sauce, balsamic vinegar, and garlic together in a bowl. Place the tilapia fillets in the mixture; allow to marinate in refrigerator at least 30 minutes.

Preheat an oven to 350 degrees F (175 degrees C). Spray a baking dish with cooking spray.

Remove tilapia from marinade, and discard the marinade. Place fillets into the prepared baking sheet, and sprinkle the black pepper over the fish.

Bake in the preheated oven until the fish flakes easily with a fork, 15 to 20 minutes.

Note:

The nutrition data for this recipe includes the full amount of the marinade Ingredients. The actual amount of the marinade consumed will vary.

Garlic Fried Rice

Things To Get

1 cup uncooked white rice

2 cups water

1 teaspoon butter

1 clove garlic, minced

1 small onion, minced

1 tablespoon lemon juice

Preparation

Combine the rice and water in a saucepan and bring to a boil. Cover, reduce heat to low, and simmer until rice is tender and water is absorbed. Set aside to cool.

Melt the butter in a large skillet over medium-high heat. Add onion and garlic; cook and stir until fragrant and lightly browned. Stir in rice and cook until coated and heated through. Remove from the heat and stir in the lemon juice.

Crispy Air Fryer Cod

Things To Get

1 pound cod, about 1-inch thick, cut into 4 pieces

¼ cup polenta

¼ cup all-purpose flour

1 ½ teaspoons seafood seasoning (such as Old Bay®)

1 ½ teaspoons garlic salt

1 teaspoon onion powder

½ teaspoon ground black pepper

½ teaspoon paprika

olive oil cooking spray

Preparation

Preheat an air fryer to 380 degrees F (195 degrees C). Pat cod pieces dry with paper towels.

Combine polenta, flour, seafood seasoning, garlic salt, onion powder, pepper, and paprika in a shallow dish. Coat each piece of cod with the breading mixture, pressing breading on each side of the fish until well coated.

Spray the basket of the air fryer with olive oil cooking spray. Arrange cod in the basket, leaving space between each piece so air can circulate. Spray the top of each piece of cod with cooking spray.

Cook for 8 minutes. Turn each piece, spray with cooking spray, and cook for 4 minutes more.

Note: :

Substitute cornmeal for the polenta, if desired.

Whiskey Chicken

Things To Get

2 skinless, boneless chicken breast halves - cut into 1/2 inch pieces

2 tablespoons soy sauce

¼ teaspoon garlic powder

1 cup pineapple juice

3 tablespoons bourbon whiskey

⅛ teaspoon ground black pepper

1 tablespoon brown sugar

Preparation

Saute chicken in a large skillet over medium high heat until cooked through (no longer pink).

In a small bowl, combine the soy sauce, garlic powder, pineapple juice, whiskey, pepper and sugar. Stir until sugar is dissolved and pour over chicken. Let simmer for 10 to 15 minutes, or until sauce is thickened to taste.

Cod with Italian Crumb Topping

Things To Get

¼ cup fine dry bread crumbs

2 tablespoons grated Parmesan cheese

1 tablespoon cornmeal

1 teaspoon olive oil

½ teaspoon Italian seasoning

⅛ teaspoon garlic powder

⅛ teaspoon ground black pepper

4 (3 ounce) fillets cod fillets

1 egg white, lightly beaten

Preparation

Preheat oven to 450 degrees F (230 degrees C).

In a small shallow bowl, stir together the bread crumbs, cheese, cornmeal, oil, italian seasoning, garlic powder and pepper; set aside.

Coat the rack of a broiling pan with cooking spray. Place the cod on the rack, folding under any thin edges of the filets. Brush with the egg white, then spoon the crumb mixture evenly on top.

Bake in a preheated oven for 10 to 12 minutes or until the fish flakes easily when tested with a fork and is opaque all the way through.

Vegan Bean Taco Filling

Things To Get

1 tablespoon olive oil

1 onion, diced

2 cloves garlic, minced

1 bell pepper, chopped

2 (14.5 ounce) cans black beans, rinsed, drained, and mashed

2 tablespoons yellow cornmeal

1 ½ tablespoons cumin

1 teaspoon paprika

1 teaspoon cayenne pepper

1 teaspoon chili powder

1 cup salsa

Preparation

Heat olive oil in a medium skillet over medium heat. Stir in onion, garlic, and bell pepper; cook until tender. Stir in mashed beans. Add the cornmeal. Mix in cumin, paprika, cayenne, chili powder, and salsa. Cover, and cook 5 minutes.

DELICIOUS AND HEALTHY DINNER RECIPES

Sheet Pan Salmon and Bell Pepper Dinner

Things To Get

2 tablespoons olive oil

4 (3 ounce) fillets salmon fillets

2 red bell peppers, chopped

1 yellow bell pepper, chopped

1 onion, sliced

Sauce:

6 tablespoons lemon juice

3 tablespoons olive oil

2 tablespoons water

1 tablespoon maple syrup

5 cloves garlic

1 ½ teaspoons salt

1 ½ teaspoons red pepper flakes

1 teaspoon ground cumin

½ bunch fresh parsley, chopped

1 lemon, sliced

Preparation

Preheat oven to 400 degrees F (200 degrees C). Grease a sheet pan with 2 tablespoons olive oil.

Place salmon fillets, red and yellow bell peppers, and onion on the prepared sheet pan.

Combine lemon juice, 3 tablespoons olive oil, water, maple syrup, garlic, salt, red pepper flakes, cumin, and parsley in a small bowl. Drizzle 2/3 of the sauce over the **Things To Get** on the sheet pan.

Bake in the preheated oven until salmon is cooked through and flakes easily with a fork, 10 to 15 minutes.

Serve with lemon slices and remaining sauce.

Turkey Spaghetti Zoodles

Things To Get

1 teaspoon extra-virgin olive oil

1 ¼ pounds ground turkey breast

1 cup diced green bell pepper

1 tablespoon minced garlic

2 teaspoons Italian seasoning

½ teaspoon ground black pepper

¼ teaspoon salt

¼ teaspoon red pepper flakes

3 cups marinara sauce

2 cups baby spinach leaves

4 zucchini, cut into noodle-shape strands

Preparation

Heat olive oil in a large skillet over medium heat. Add turkey breast, green pepper, garlic, Italian seasoning, ground black pepper, salt, and red pepper flakes; cook and stir until turkey is lightly browned, 4 to 5 minutes.

Stir marinara sauce and baby spinach into the turkey mixture; cook and stir until marinara sauce is warm through, about 3 minutes.

Stir zucchini noodles into the sauce with tongs; cook and stir until the zucchini is slightly tender, 2 to 3 minutes.

Note: :

I use an organic, no salt added, low sugar marinara sauce. To make the zucchini noodles, use a spiralizer or vegetable peeler.

Spinach Whole Wheat Quesadillas

Things To Get

2 (10 inch) whole wheat tortillas

3 cups fresh spinach leaves

⅔cup shredded Cheddar cheese

1 green onion, chopped

½ teaspoon garlic powder

½ teaspoon chili powder

Preparation

Heat a large non-stick skillet over medium-high heat. Place 1 tortilla onto the skillet. Sprinkle about half the Cheddar cheese evenly over the tortilla.

Top with the spinach, green onions, garlic powder, and chili powder. Cover with the remaining Cheddar cheese. Place the second tortilla on top.

Cook until the bottom tortilla starts to develop a bit of color and starts to crisp, about 3 minutes. To flip and cook the other side, slide the quesadilla off the non-stick pan onto a dinner plate, cover with another dinner plate and flip. The crispy tortilla side should now be on top. Slide the quesadilla back onto the pan and cook until the bottom tortilla starts turning crisp, about 3 minutes more. Slide onto a cutting board, and cut into 8 wedges to serve.

Jack's Old-Fashioned Beef and Vegetable Soup

Things To Get

2 tablespoons butter

1 onion, coarsely chopped

4 stalks celery, chopped

⅓ pound lean round steak, cut into 1/2-inch cubes

1 quart beef stock

1 quart water

1 bay leaf

¼ teaspoon dried marjoram

¼ teaspoon dried oregano

2 pounds beef soup bones

1 large potato, peeled and cut into large chunks

1 large carrot, peeled and cut into large chunks

1 small green bell pepper, chopped

¼ cup dry black beans

¼ cup dried split peas

¼ cup white rice

¼ cup elbow macaroni

1 cup crushed tomatoes in puree

¼ cup chopped cabbage

1 cup red wine

salt and ground black pepper to taste

Preparation

Melt the butter in a large stockpot over medium heat; cook the onion, celery, and steak in the melted butter until the onions caramelize, 7 to 10 minutes. Add the beef stock, water, bay leaf, marjoram, oregano, and soup bones; lower the heat to medium-low and simmer 3 hours, skimming froth off the top of the soup as it develops.

Add the potato, carrot, bell pepper, black beans, split peas, rice, macaroni, tomatoes in puree, cabbage, and red wine to the stockpot. Simmer 1 hour more. Remove the soup bones, scraping any meat from them back into the pot. Season with salt and pepper to serve.

Pork Stir Fry

Things To Get

5 tablespoons reduced-sodium soy sauce

2 tablespoons rice wine vinegar

1 tablespoon cornstarch

2 tablespoons sesame oil, divided

1 (1 pound) pork tenderloin, cut into strips

1 fresh red chile pepper, chopped

2 cloves garlic, minced

1 onion, chopped

1 green bell pepper, chopped

1 head bok choy, leaves and stalks separated, chopped

2 crowns broccoli, chopped

1 teaspoon ground ginger

Preparation

Whisk soy sauce, vinegar, and cornstarch together in a small bowl; set aside.

Heat 1 tablespoon sesame oil in a wok over medium-high heat. Cook and stir tenderloin strips in hot oil until just browned, 2 to 4 minutes. Transfer pork to a plate and return the wok to heat.

Add remaining sesame oil to the wok; cook and stir red chile pepper and garlic in hot oil until sizzling, 15 to 30 seconds. Add onion and bell pepper; cook and stir until onion starts to soften, 2 to 3 minutes.

Stir chopped bok choy stalks into onion mixture; cook and stir until stems begin to soften, about 3 minutes.

Add broccoli to the wok; cook and stir until slightly softened, about 2 minutes. Add pork, chopped bok choy leaves, and soy sauce mixture; cook and stir until well-combined. Season pork mixture with ginger; cook and stir until bok choy leaves start to wilt and broccoli is tender, 5 to 7 minutes.

Quick Fish Tacos

Things To Get

¼ cup reduced-fat sour cream

2 tablespoons lime juice

salt and ground black pepper to taste

1 jalapeno pepper, halved lengthwise

2 ½ cups shredded red cabbage

4 green onions, thinly sliced

2 tablespoons olive oil

1 pound tilapia fillets, cut into strips

8 (6 inch) flour tortillas

½ cup chopped fresh cilantro

Preparation

Mix sour cream and lime juice together in a large bowl; season with salt and black pepper. Reserve about half the mixture in another bowl for serving. Mince half the jalapeno pepper; save other half for later. Toss cabbage, green onions, and minced jalapeno half in remaining sour cream mixture until slaw is well mixed.

Heat olive oil and remaining jalapeno half in a large skillet over medium heat; swirl oil to coat skillet evenly. Season tilapia fillets with salt and pepper. Pan-fry fish strips in the skillet in 2 batches until fish is golden brown and easily flaked with a fork, 5 to 6 minutes. Discard jalapeno half.

Heat tortillas in the microwave on high until warm, 20 to 30 seconds.

Serve fish in warmed tortillas topped with cabbage slaw, reserved sour cream mixture, and cilantro.

One-Skillet Mexican Quinoa

Things To Get

1 tablespoon olive oil

1 medium jalapeño pepper, chopped

2 cloves garlic, chopped

1 (15 ounce) can black beans, rinsed and drained

1 (14.5 ounce) can fire-roasted diced tomatoes

1 cup yellow corn

1 cup quinoa

1 cup chicken broth

1 tablespoon red pepper flakes, or to taste

1 ½ teaspoons chili powder

½ teaspoon ground cumin

kosher salt and ground black pepper to taste

1 medium avocado - peeled, pitted, and diced

1 medium lime, juiced

2 tablespoons chopped fresh cilantro

Preparation

Heat oil in a large skillet over medium-high heat. Sauté jalapeño pepper and garlic in the hot oil until fragrant, about 1 minute.

Stir black beans, tomatoes, corn, quinoa, and chicken broth into the skillet. Season with pepper flakes, chili powder, cumin, salt, and black pepper; bring to a boil.

Cover the skillet with a lid, reduce heat to low, and simmer until quinoa is tender and liquid is mostly absorbed, about 20 minutes.

Add avocado, lime juice, and cilantro; stir until combined.

Roasted Balsamic Chicken with Baby Tomatoes

Things To Get

½ cup balsamic vinegar

1 tablespoon olive oil

1 tablespoon Dijon mustard, or more to taste

1 clove garlic, or more to taste, minced

salt and freshly ground pepper to taste

4 large skinless, boneless chicken breast halves

1 pint cherry tomatoes, halved

1 lemon, zested and juiced

Preparation

Mix balsamic vinegar, olive oil, mustard, and garlic together in an oven-safe baking dish; season with salt and pepper. Place the chicken breasts in the vinegar mixture.

Marinate chicken in the refrigerator for at least 4 hours.

Preheat oven to 400 degrees F (200 degrees C).

Roast chicken in the preheated oven for about 30 minutes. Add tomatoes to the baking dish and continue cooking until the chicken is no longer pink in the center and the juices run clear, about 10 minutes more. An instant-read thermometer inserted into the center should read at least 165 degrees F (74 degrees C).

Sprinkle lemon zest and drizzle lemon juice over the chicken.

Hamburger Steak with Onions and Gravy

Things To Get

1 pound ground beef

¼ cup bread crumbs

1 egg

1 teaspoon Worcestershire sauce

½ teaspoon seasoned salt

½ teaspoon onion powder

½ teaspoon garlic powder

⅛ teaspoon ground black pepper

1 tablespoon vegetable oil

1 cup thinly sliced onion

2 tablespoons all-purpose flour

1 cup beef broth

1 tablespoon cooking sherry

½ teaspoon seasoned salt

Preparation

Mix ground beef, bread crumbs, egg, Worcestershire sauce, salt, onion powder, garlic powder, and pepper together in a large bowl until combined. Form into 8 balls and flatten into patties.

Heat oil in a large skillet over medium heat. Add patties and onion; fry until patties are nicely browned, about 4 minutes per side. Transfer beef patties to a plate, and keep warm.

Sprinkle flour over onions and drippings in the skillet. Stir in flour with a fork, scraping bits of beef off of the bottom of the skillet as you stir. Gradually mix in beef broth and sherry. Season with seasoned salt. Simmer and stir over medium-low heat until gravy thickens, about 5 minutes.

Reduce heat to low, return patties to the gravy, cover, and simmer until cooked through, about 15 minutes.

Shrimp Saute on Cauliflower Rice

Things To Get

½ head cauliflower

1 teaspoon olive oil, or as needed

1 cup chicken stock, divided

1 tablespoon ground cumin

salt and ground black pepper to taste

1 lime, juiced, divided

2 tablespoons coconut oil, or as needed

20 baby bella mushrooms, diced

2 Fresno peppers, diced

1 onion, diced

1 large tomato, diced

3 tablespoons almond flour

1 tablespoon garlic powder

1 tablespoon chili powder

1 tablespoon dried oregano

½ tablespoon dried tarragon

3 cups fresh spinach

1 pound large shrimp, peeled and deveined

Preparation

Put cauliflower into the bowl of a food processor and pulse until the consistency is like white rice. Transfer cauliflower to a skillet over medium-low heat. Add olive oil and 1/2 cup chicken stock. When cauliflower is warm, about 5 minutes, add cumin, salt, black pepper, and juice of 1/2 a lime. Cover and allow cauliflower rice to steam until tender but slightly firm while you prepare the shrimp saute.

Heat coconut oil in a separate skillet over medium heat. Add mushrooms, Fresno peppers, onion, and tomato. Toss and season with salt and black pepper. Cook until vegetables are soft and mushrooms release moisture, 5 to 10 minutes. Add almond flour and stir to create a pasty roux; cook for 1 to 2 minutes. Pour in remaining chicken stock slowly until desired consistency.

Bring sauce to a simmer, about 5 minutes. Add garlic powder, chili powder, oregano, and tarragon. Season with salt and black pepper to taste. Add remaining lime juice and stir to combine. Mix in spinach and cook just until wilted, about 1 minute. Stir in shrimp and immediately remove skillet from heat to avoid overcooking.

Top cauliflower rice with shrimp saute.

Note:

You can use 4 garlic cloves in place of the garlic powder.

Chicken Vegetable Barley Soup

Things To Get

1 cup slivered almonds

2 tablespoons olive oil

1 medium onion, chopped

1 cup chopped celery

4 cups sliced fresh mushrooms

4 cloves garlic, minced

1 cup chopped carrots

5 cups diced red potatoes

3 cups chopped cooked chicken

2 ½ quarts chicken broth

1 cup quick-cooking barley

2 tablespoons butter

½ cup chopped fresh parsley

salt and black pepper to taste

Preparation

Preheat oven to 400 degrees F (200 degrees C). Spread slivered almonds evenly over a baking sheet. Toast in preheated oven until golden brown and fragrant.

Heat the oil in a large stock pot over medium heat. Cook onions, celery, mushrooms, and garlic in oil until onions are tender.

Stir in carrots, potatoes, chicken, and broth. Bring to a boil, then stir in barley. Reduce heat, cover, and simmer 20 minutes.

Remove from heat, and stir in butter, parsley, and toasted almonds. Season with salt and pepper to taste.

Easy Baked Tilapia

Things To Get

4 (4 ounce) fillets tilapia

2 teaspoons butter

½ teaspoon garlic salt, or to taste

¼ teaspoon seafood seasoning (such as Old Bay®), or to taste

1 lemon, sliced

1 (16 ounce) package frozen cauliflower with broccoli and red pepper

salt and ground black pepper to taste

Preparation

Preheat the oven to 375 degrees F (190 degrees F). Grease a 9x13-inch baking dish.

Place tilapia fillets in the bottom of the baking dish, then dot with butter and season with garlic salt and seafood seasoning. Top each fillet with a slice or two of lemon. Arrange frozen mixed vegetables around fillets and season lightly with salt and pepper. Cover the dish with aluminum foil.

Bake in the preheated oven until vegetables are tender and fish flakes easily with a fork, 25 to 30 minutes.

Black Beans and Rice

Things To Get

1 teaspoon olive oil

1 onion, chopped

2 cloves garlic, minced

¾ cup uncooked white rice

1 ½ cups low sodium, low fat vegetable broth

3 ½ cups canned black beans, drained

1 teaspoon ground cumin

¼ teaspoon cayenne pepper

Preparation

Heat oil in a saucepan over medium-high heat. Add onion and garlic; cook and stir until onion has softened, about 4 minutes. Stir in rice to coat; cook and stir for 2 minutes.

Add vegetable broth and bring to a boil. Cover, reduce to a simmer, and cook until liquid is absorbed, about 20 minutes.

Stir in beans, cumin, and cayenne; cook until beans are warmed through.

Tomato and Garlic Pasta

Things To Get

2 pounds tomatoes

1 (8 ounce) package angel hair pasta

1 tablespoon olive oil, or as needed

4 cloves crushed garlic

1 tablespoon tomato paste

salt to taste

ground black pepper to taste

1 tablespoon chopped fresh basil

¼ cup grated Parmesan cheese

Preparation

Place tomatoes in a large pot and cover with cold
water. Bring just to a boil. Pour off water, and cover

again with cold water. Peel the skin off tomatoes and cut into small pieces.

Bring a large pot of lightly salted water to a boil. Cook angel hair pasta in the boiling water, stirring occasionally, until tender yet firm to the bite, 4 to 5 minutes.

Meanwhile, heat olive oil in a large skillet or pan, making sure there is enough to cover the bottom of the pan, and sauté garlic until opaque but not browned. Stir in tomato paste. Immediately stir in the tomatoes, salt, and pepper. Reduce heat, and simmer until pasta is ready, adding basil at the end.

Drain pasta, do not rinse in cold water. Toss with a bit of olive oil, then mix into the sauce.

Reduce heat as low as possible. Keep warm, uncovered, for about 10 minutes when it is ready to serve. Garnish generously with fresh Parmesan cheese.

Tips

There are many variations to try for this pasta. A few favorite examples: sauté fresh quartered mushrooms with the garlic, or add shoestring zucchini along with the tomato.

Wonton Soup

Things To Get

Wontons:

½ pound boneless pork loin, coarsely chopped

2 ounces peeled shrimp, finely chopped

1 tablespoon Chinese rice wine

1 tablespoon light soy sauce

1 teaspoon brown sugar

1 teaspoon finely chopped green onions

1 teaspoon chopped fresh ginger root

24 (3.5 inch square) wonton wrappers

Soup:

3 cups chicken stock

2 tablespoons finely chopped green onions

Preparation

Make the wontons: Mix pork, shrimp, rice wine, soy sauce, brown sugar, green onions, and ginger together in a large bowl until well combined. Let stand for 25 to 30 minutes.

Spoon about 1 teaspoon filling onto the center of a wonton wrapper. Moisten all four wrapper edges with water and fold over filling to make a triangle; press the edges firmly to seal. Bring left and right corners together above filling; overlap the tips of these corners, moisten with water, and press together to seal. Repeat until all wrappers have been filled and sealed.

Make the soup: Bring chicken stock to a rolling boil in a pot. Gently drop in wontons and cook for 5 minutes.

Ladle into bowls and garnish with green onions.

Fish Tacos

Things To Get

Beer Batter:

1 cup all-purpose flour

2 tablespoons cornstarch

1 teaspoon baking powder

½ teaspoon salt

1 cup beer

1 egg

White Sauce:

½ cup plain yogurt

½ cup mayonnaise

1 lime, juiced

1 jalapeno pepper, minced

1 teaspoon minced capers

1 teaspoon ground cayenne pepper

½ teaspoon dried oregano

½ teaspoon ground cumin

½ teaspoon dried dill weed

Fish Tacos:

1 quart oil for frying

1 pound cod fillets, cut into 2 to 3 ounce portions

2 tablespoons all-purpose flour, or more as needed

1 (12 ounce) package corn tortillas

½ medium head cabbage, finely shredded

Preparation

Make beer batter: Combine flour, cornstarch, baking powder, and salt in a large bowl. Blend beer and egg in a separate bowl, then quickly stir into flour mixture until combined with a few lumps remaining.

Make white sauce: Mix together yogurt and mayonnaise in a medium bowl. Gradually stir in fresh lime juice until consistency is slightly runny. Season with jalapeño, capers, cayenne, oregano, cumin, and dill.

Start fish tacos: Heat oil in a deep-fryer to 375 degrees F (190 degrees C).

Dust fish pieces lightly with flour. Dip into beer batter, then fry in hot oil until crisp and golden brown. Drain on paper towels.

Lightly fry tortillas in hot oil until just crisped, but not too crisp. Drain on paper towels.

Place fried fish in tortillas; top with shredded cabbage and white sauce.

Chana Masala (Savory Indian Chick Peas)

Things To Get

1 onion, chopped

1 tomato, chopped

1 (1 inch) piece fresh ginger, peeled and chopped

4 cloves garlic, chopped, or more to taste

1 green chile pepper, seeded and chopped (Optional)

3 tablespoons olive oil

2 fresh bay leaves

1 teaspoon chili powder

1 teaspoon coriander powder

1 teaspoon garam masala

½ teaspoon turmeric powder

1 pinch salt to taste

water as needed

1 (15 ounce) can chickpeas

1 teaspoon fresh cilantro leaves, for garnish, or more to taste

Preparation

Grind onion, tomato, ginger, garlic, and chile pepper together in a food processor into a paste.

Heat olive oil in a large skillet over medium heat. Fry bay leaves in hot oil until fragrant, about 30 seconds. Pour the paste into the skillet and cook until the oil begins to separate from the mixture and is golden brown in color, 2 to 3 minutes. Season the mixture with chili powder, coriander, gram masala, turmeric, and salt; cook and stir until very hot, 2 to 3 minutes.

Stir enough water into the mixture to get a thick gravy; bring to a boil and stir chickpeas into the gravy. Reduce heat to medium and cook until the chickpeas are heated through, 5 to 7 minutes. Garnish with cilantro.

Note:

Serve with a 'Mattar Paneer' recipe to round out this Indian dinner.

As an optional serving suggestion, use the "Indian Naan Bread" recipe instead of rice as a companion to this dish.

Parchment Baked Salmon

Things To Get

1 (8 ounce) salmon fillet

salt and ground black pepper to taste

¼ cup chopped basil leaves

olive oil cooking spray

1 lemon, thinly sliced

Preparation

Preheat the oven to 400 degrees F (200 degrees C). Move an oven rack to the lowest position.

Place salmon fillet, skin-side down, in the middle of a large piece of parchment paper; season with salt and black pepper. Cut two 3-inch slits into fillet with a sharp knife. Stuff chopped basil leaves into the slits. Spray fillet with cooking spray and arrange lemon slices on top.

Fold the edges of parchment paper over fillet several times to seal it into an airtight packet. Place sealed packet onto a baking sheet.

Bake in the preheated oven on the bottom rack until salmon flakes easily and flesh is pink and opaque with an interior of slightly darker pink color, about 25 minutes. An instant-read thermometer inserted into the thickest part of fillet should read at least 145 degrees F (65 degrees C). To serve, cut open the parchment paper and remove lemon slices before plating.

Parchment Baked Salmon

Things To Get

1 (8 ounce) salmon fillet

salt and ground black pepper to taste

¼ cup chopped basil leaves

olive oil cooking spray

1 lemon, thinly sliced

Preparation

Preheat the oven to 400 degrees F (200 degrees C). Move an oven rack to the lowest position.

Place salmon fillet, skin-side down, in the middle of a large piece of parchment paper; season with salt and black pepper. Cut two 3-inch slits into fillet with a sharp knife. Stuff chopped basil leaves into the slits. Spray fillet with cooking spray and arrange lemon slices on top.

Fold the edges of parchment paper over fillet several times to seal it into an airtight packet. Place sealed packet onto a baking sheet.

Bake in the preheated oven on the bottom rack until salmon flakes easily and flesh is pink and opaque with an interior of slightly darker pink color, about 25 minutes. An instant-read thermometer inserted into the thickest part of fillet should read at least 145 degrees F (65 degrees C). To serve, cut open the parchment paper and remove lemon slices before plating.

Muesli

Things To Get

4 ½ cups rolled oats

1 cup raisins

½ cup toasted wheat germ

½ cup wheat bran

½ cup oat bran

½ cup chopped walnuts

¼ cup packed brown sugar

¼ cup raw sunflower seeds

Preparation

Combine oats, raisins, wheat germ, wheat bran, oat bran, walnuts, brown sugar, and sunflower seeds in a large bowl; mix well. Store muesli in an airtight container at room temperature for up to 2 months.

Lemon-Orange Orange Roughy

Things To Get

1 tablespoon olive oil

4 (4 ounce) fillets orange roughy

1 orange, juiced

1 lemon, juiced

½ teaspoon lemon pepper

Preparation

Heat oil in a large skillet over medium-high heat.

Place fillets into hot oil. Drizzle with orange juice and lemon juice, then sprinkle fillets with lemon pepper. Cook until fish flakes easily with a fork, 2 to 3 minutes per side. An instant-read thermometer inserted into the center should read at least 145 degrees F (63 degrees C).

Healthier Stuffed Peppers

Things To Get

1 cup water

½ cup brown rice

1 pound lean ground beef

1 onion, chopped

2 cloves garlic, minced

2 green bell peppers

2 red bell peppers

2 yellow bell peppers

2 (8 ounce) cans natural tomato sauce

1 tablespoon Worcestershire sauce

salt and ground black pepper to taste

1 teaspoon Italian seasoning

¼ cup grated Parmesan cheese, optional

Preparation

Preheat the oven to 350 degrees F (175 degrees C).

Bring water and brown rice to a boil in a saucepan. Reduce heat to medium-low, cover, and simmer until rice is tender and liquid is absorbed, 45 to 50 minutes.

Meanwhile, warm a large skillet over medium heat. Add beef, onion, and garlic to the hot skillet; cook and stir until meat is evenly browned and onion is softened, about 5 minutes. Set aside.

Remove and discard tops, seeds, and membranes of green, red, and yellow bell peppers. Arrange peppers in a baking dish with the hollowed sides facing upward. Slice the bottoms off peppers if necessary so that they stand upright.

Mix browned beef, cooked rice, 1 can tomato sauce, Worcestershire sauce, salt, and pepper in a bowl. Spoon mixture into each hollowed pepper. Mix remaining tomato sauce with Italian seasoning in a bowl; pour over peppers.

Bake in the preheated oven, basting with sauce every 15 minutes, until peppers are tender, about 1 hour. Sprinkle peppers with grated Parmesan cheese; serve warm.

Note:

This recipe is a healthier version of Sausage and Rice Stuffed Peppers.

Linguine with White Clam Sauce

Things To Get

1 (12 ounce) package linguine pasta

¼ cup olive oil

1 clove garlic, minced

3 (8 ounce) cans minced clams, with juice

¾ cup chopped parsley

2 tablespoons white wine

1 teaspoon dried basil

½ teaspoon salt

Preparation

Bring a large pot of lightly salted water to a boil. Cook linguine at a boil until tender yet firm to the bite, about 10 minutes.

Meanwhile, heat olive oil in a large skillet over medium heat. Add garlic; cook and stir until fragrant, about 1 minute. Stir in liquid from clams, parsley, white wine, basil, and salt; simmer for 10 minutes.

Stir in clams until heated through. Add cooked linguine pasta; toss to combine and serve warm.

Ginger Glazed Mahi Mahi

Things To Get

3 tablespoons honey

3 tablespoons soy sauce

3 tablespoons balsamic vinegar

2 teaspoons olive oil

1 teaspoon grated fresh ginger root

1 clove garlic, crushed or to taste

4 (6 ounce) mahi mahi fillets

salt and pepper to taste

1 tablespoon vegetable oil

Preparation

Mix honey, soy sauce, balsamic vinegar, olive oil, ginger, and garlic together in a shallow dish. Season fish fillets with salt and pepper; place them skin-sides down in the dish with marinade. Cover and refrigerate for 20 minutes.

Heat vegetable oil in a large skillet over medium-high heat. Remove fish fillets, reserving marinade. Fry fish for 4 to 6 minutes on each side, turning only once, until fish flakes easily with a fork. Remove fillets to a serving platter and keep warm.

Pour reserved marinade into the skillet; simmer over medium heat until reduced to a glaze. Spoon glaze over fish and serve.

DELICIOUS AND HEALTHY SOUP AND STEW RECIPES

Dry Onion Soup Mix

Things To Get

¼ cup dried onion flakes

2 tablespoons low-sodium beef bouillon granules

¼ teaspoon onion powder

¼ teaspoon parsley flakes

⅛ teaspoon celery seed

⅛ teaspoon paprika

⅛ teaspoon ground black pepper

Preparation

Stir onion flakes, beef bouillon granules, onion powder, parsley flakes, celery seed, paprika, and black pepper together in a bowl.

Use as a substitute for a 1-ounce envelope of dry onion soup mix.

Note:

To make this into soup, bring 3 1/2 cups water to a boil in a medium saucepan. Whisk in soup mix, reduce heat to low, and simmer for 5 minutes.

Quick and Easy Vegetable Soup

Things To Get

1 (14.5 ounce) can diced tomatoes

1 (14 ounce) can chicken broth

1 (11.5 ounce) can tomato-vegetable juice cocktail

2 carrots, sliced

2 stalks celery, diced

1 large potato, diced

1 cup chopped fresh green beans

1 cup fresh corn kernels

1 cup water

salt and pepper to taste

1 pinch Creole seasoning, or more to taste

Preparation

Combine tomatoes, chicken broth, tomato juice, carrots, celery, potato, green beans, corn, and water in a large stockpot. Season with salt, pepper, and Creole seasoning.

Bring to a boil over medium heat and simmer until vegetables are tender, about 30 minutes.

Easy Chinese Corn Soup

Things To Get

1 (15 ounce) can cream style corn

1 (14.5 ounce) can low-sodium chicken broth

1 tablespoon cornstarch

2 tablespoons water

1 large egg, beaten

Preparation

Combine corn and chicken broth in a saucepan. Bring to a boil over medium-high heat.

Mix together cornstarch and water in a small bowl or cup; pour into the boiling corn soup, and continue cooking for about 2 minutes, or until thickened.

Gradually add beaten egg while stirring the soup. Remove from heat and serve.

Maryland Crab Soup

Things To Get

2 (14.5 ounce) cans stewed tomatoes

3 cups water

2 cups beef broth

1 cup fresh lima beans

1 cup frozen corn kernels

1 cup sliced carrots

2 tablespoons chopped onion

2 tablespoons Old Bay Seasoning TM

1 gallon water

10 blue crab claws, steamed (Optional)

1 pound blue crab crabmeat

Preparation

Place stewed tomatoes, 3 cups water, beef broth, lima beans, corn, sliced carrots, chopped onion, and Old Bay seasoning in a 4-quart pot. Bring to a simmer over medium heat; cover and cook for 5 minutes.

Bring 1 gallon water to a boil in a large pot. Add crab claws and boil for 6 minutes; drain.

Stir crabmeat and boiled crab claws into tomato and vegetable mixture. Cover and simmer for 10 to 15 minutes. Serve hot.

Instant Pot Beef Bone Broth

Things To Get

cooking spray

2 pounds frozen beef bones

2 carrots, chopped

2 stalks celery, chopped

1 medium onion, quartered

5 cloves garlic, whole

6 cups boiling water

2 bay leaves

1 tablespoon apple cider vinegar

1 teaspoon sea salt

10 whole black peppercorns

Preparation

Preheat the oven to 400 degrees F (200 degrees C). Line a baking sheet with aluminum foil and spray with cooking spray.

Place beef bones, carrots, celery, onion, and garlic on the prepared baking sheet.

Roast in the preheated oven until browned, about 45 minutes.

Scrape roasted bones and vegetables into a multi-functional pressure cooker (such as Instant Pot). Add boiling water, bay leaves, vinegar, sea salt, and peppercorns. Close and lock the lid. Select Manual function according to manufacturer's instructions;

set timer for 120 minutes. Allow 10 to 15 minutes for pressure to build.

Release pressure using the natural-release method according to manufacturer's instructions, 10 to 40 minutes. Unlock and remove the lid. Remove bones and vegetables and discard. Line a strainer with cheesecloth and set over a large bowl. Pour broth through the strainer and discard solids.

Allow broth to cool. Remove and discard the fat layer.

Tips

I use bones from roasts and grilled steak, but do not use bones that have BBQ sauce on them.

Canadian Yellow Split Pea Soup with Ham

Things To Get

1 ham bone with some meat

2 ½ cups yellow split peas

5 stalks celery, diced

4 carrots, diced

½ large Spanish onion, diced

2 tablespoons kosher salt

2 teaspoons dried thyme

1 bay leaf (Optional)

1 pinch ground black pepper, or to taste

8 cups water, or as needed

Preparation

Place ham bone, split peas, celery, carrots, onion, salt, thyme, bay leaf, and pepper into a large pot; pour in water. Bring mixture to a boil and skim off any foam with a spoon.

Reduce the heat and place a lid on the pot, slightly ajar to allow some evaporation. Simmer, stirring occasionally, until peas are tender and soup is thick, about 3 hours.

Remove ham bone from soup; remove meat from ham bone, chop, and return to the pot.

Tips

You can substitute 2 smoked pork hocks or 1 small ham shank for the leftover ham bone. Adjust the thickness of the soup by adding a little water to thin it, or remove broth with a spoon to thicken it up. I sometimes use an immersion blender for a quick second to blend the soup, making sure to leave some chunky peas, carrots, celery, and ham.

Classic Turkey and Rice Soup

Things To Get

Stock:

1 turkey carcass

1 large onion, halved and skin left on

1 large carrot, roughly chopped

1 stalk celery, roughly chopped

1 head garlic, halved

1 teaspoon dried rosemary

1 teaspoon dried thyme

2 bay leaves

salt and ground black pepper to taste

2 quarts water, or as needed

Soup:

2 large onions, diced

2 carrots, diced

2 stalks celery, diced

2 cloves garlic, minced

1 teaspoon poultry seasoning

1 teaspoon dried rosemary

1 teaspoon onion powder

2 cups cooked rice

salt and ground black pepper to taste

Preparation

Make stock: Combine turkey carcass, onion, carrot, celery, garlic, rosemary, thyme, bay leaves, salt, and pepper in a stockpot; pour in enough water to cover. Bring mixture to a boil, cover the pot, reduce heat, and simmer until flavors have blended, about 1 hour.

Remove turkey carcass and pull remaining meat from bones; reserve meat and discard carcass. Use a slotted spoon to remove and discard vegetables and bay leaves.

Make soup: Stir onions, carrots, celery, garlic, poultry seasoning, rosemary, and onion powder into stock; bring to a boil. Reduce heat, cover the pot, and simmer until vegetables are very tender, 20 to 30 minutes.

Add cooked rice and reserved turkey meat to soup; season with salt and pepper. Cook until rice and turkey meat are warmed through, about 5 minutes.

Tips

You can use turkey meat instead of a carcass. Roast legs or thighs in the oven, then continue with instructions for the stock. To further reduce fat, make the stock ahead and chill it in the refrigerator. Any fat will rise to the top and can be easily removed.

Hearty Vegan Slow-Cooker Chili

Things To Get

1 tablespoon olive oil

2 onions, chopped

1 green bell pepper, chopped

1 red bell pepper, chopped

1 yellow bell pepper, chopped

4 cloves garlic, minced

2 (14.5 ounce) cans diced tomatoes with juice

1 (15 ounce) can black beans, rinsed and drained

1 (15 ounce) can garbanzo beans, drained

1 (15 ounce) can kidney beans, rinsed and drained

2 (6 ounce) cans tomato paste

1 (10 ounce) package frozen chopped spinach, thawed and drained

1 cup frozen corn kernels, thawed

1 zucchini, chopped

1 yellow squash, chopped

6 tablespoons chili powder

1 tablespoon ground cumin

1 tablespoon dried oregano

1 tablespoon dried parsley

½ teaspoon salt

½ teaspoon ground black pepper

1 (8 ounce) can tomato sauce, or more if needed

1 cup vegetable broth, or more if needed

Preparation

Heat olive oil in a large skillet over medium heat. Add onions, bell peppers, and garlic; cook and stir until onions start to brown, 8 to 10 minutes.

Transfer mixture into a slow cooker. Stir in tomatoes, black beans, garbanzo beans, kidney beans, tomato paste, spinach, corn, zucchini, yellow squash, chili powder, cumin, oregano, parsley, salt, and pepper until thoroughly mixed. Pour the tomato sauce and vegetable broth over the Ingredients.

Cook on Low for 4 to 5 hours. Check seasoning. If chili is too thick, add more tomato sauce and vegetable broth to desired thickness. Cook on Low for an additional 1 to 2 hours.

Vegan Split Pea Soup

Things To Get

1 tablespoon vegetable oil

1 onion, chopped

3 cloves garlic, minced

1 bay leaf

7 ½ cups water

2 cups dried split peas

½ cup barley

1 ½ teaspoons salt

3 potatoes, diced

3 carrots, chopped

3 stalks celery, chopped

½ cup chopped parsley

½ teaspoon dried basil

½ teaspoon dried thyme

½ teaspoon ground black pepper

Preparation

Heat oil in a large pot over medium-high heat. Sauté onion, garlic, and bay leaf in hot oil until onions are translucent, about 5 minutes. Add water, peas, barley, and salt; bring to a boil. Reduce heat to low and simmer for 2 hours, stirring occasionally.

Add potatoes, carrots, celery, parsley, basil, thyme, and pepper. Simmer until peas and vegetables are tender, about 1 hour.

Chicken, Rice, and Vegetable Soup

Things To Get

5 cups water, or more as needed, divided

1 (14.5 ounce) can chicken broth

2 skinless, boneless chicken breast halves - cut into cubes

3 medium carrots, chopped

3 stalks celery, chopped

1 medium onion, chopped

2 cubes chicken bouillon

⅓cup uncooked white rice

salt and pepper to taste

Preparation

Combine 4 cups water and chicken broth in a large saucepan over high heat; bring to a boil. Add chicken, carrots, celery, onion, and bouillon cubes. Reduce the heat to low, cover, and simmer until vegetables are tender, about 15 minutes.

Add rice and up to 1 cup water if necessary; simmer until rice is tender, about 15 minutes. Season with salt and pepper.

Beaker's Vegetable Barley Soup

Things To Get

2 quarts vegetable broth

1 (15 ounce) can garbanzo beans, drained

1 (14.5 ounce) can diced tomatoes with juice

1 cup uncooked barley

2 large carrots, chopped

2 stalks celery, chopped

1 onion, chopped

1 zucchini, chopped

3 bay leaves

1 teaspoon garlic powder

1 teaspoon white sugar

1 teaspoon salt

1 teaspoon dried parsley

1 teaspoon curry powder

1 teaspoon paprika

1 teaspoon Worcestershire sauce

½ teaspoon ground black pepper

Preparation

Pour broth into a large pot. Add beans, tomatoes with juice, barley, carrots, celery, onion, zucchini, and bay leaves. Season with garlic powder, sugar, salt, parsley, curry powder, paprika, Worcestershire sauce, and pepper. Bring to a boil, then reduce heat.

Cover and simmer for 1 1/2 hours. Remove bay leaves before serving.

Tips

The soup will be very thick. You may adjust by adding more broth or less barley if desired.

Beef Bone Broth

Things To Get

3 ½ pounds beef bones, such as oxtail, short rib, knuckle, and shank

2 stalks celery, cut into 2-inch pieces

1 large onion, cut into 8 pieces

1 medium leek - roots trimmed off, cleaned, and cut into 2-inch pieces

1 whole head garlic, halved crosswise

12 cups water, or as needed

2 bay leaves, or more to taste

1 tablespoon white vinegar

1 teaspoon salt

1 teaspoon ground black pepper

Preparation

Preheat the oven to 450 degrees F (230 degrees C). Line a baking sheet with aluminum foil.

Place beef bones on the prepared baking sheet.

Roast bones in the preheated oven for 40 minutes, turning over at the halfway point.

Carefully place bones into a large stockpot and pour in any juices that have collected on the baking sheet. Add celery, onion, leek, and garlic to the stockpot, and add just enough water to completely cover the bones. Stir in bay leaves, vinegar, salt, and pepper.

Bring broth to a boil over medium-high heat. Reduce heat to a very low simmer and cover, venting the lid a bit. Simmer for 12 hours, occasionally skimming off any foam and "gunk" that rises to the top. Add additional water whenever bones and vegetables are no longer covered.

Remove the pot from the heat and cool broth to room temperature. Strain broth with a fine-mesh strainer into a clean pot. Discard bones and vegetables.

Note: :

Use a mix of bones, such as oxtail or short ribs, because these are marrow bones or bones that may have some meat on them.

Shrimp Stock

Things To Get

shrimp shells from 2 pounds of shrimp, or to taste

½ cup roughly chopped onion

¼ cup roughly chopped celery

¼ cup celery leaves, or to taste

1 medium lemon, sliced

2 cloves garlic, crushed

1 teaspoon whole black peppercorns

3 sprigs fresh thyme

2 large bay leaves

8 cups cold water

Preparation

Combine shrimp shells, onion, celery, celery leaves, lemon, garlic, peppercorns, thyme sprigs, and bay leaves in a saucepan. Pour in water and bring to a boil over medium-high heat. Reduce the heat to low and simmer until reduced by half, skimming off foam as necessary, 45 minutes to 1 hour.

Strain and discard solids. Use immediately, or let cool to room temperature and refrigerate or freeze for later use.

DELICIOUS AND HEALTHY SALAD RECIPES

Crab Ceviche

Things To Get

1 (8 ounce) package imitation crabmeat, flaked

1 tablespoon olive oil

2 large tomatoes, chopped

3 serrano peppers, finely chopped

1 red onion, finely chopped

½ bunch cilantro, chopped

2 limes, juiced

salt and pepper to taste

Preparation

Place imitation crab into a large glass or porcelain bowl; stir in olive oil until well coated. Stir in tomatoes, serrano peppers, onion, and cilantro. Squeeze lime juice on top and mix well. Season generously with salt and pepper. Cover and refrigerate for about 1 hour before serving.

Grilled Corn Salad

Things To Get

6 ears freshly shucked corn

1 medium green bell pepper, diced

2 medium Roma (plum) tomatoes, diced

¼ cup diced red onion

½ bunch fresh cilantro, chopped, or more to taste

2 teaspoons olive oil, or to taste

salt and ground black pepper to taste

Preparation

Preheat an outdoor grill for medium heat and lightly oil the grate.

Roast corn on the preheated grill, turning occasionally, until tender and specks of black appear, about 10 minutes. Remove from the grill and let sit until just cool enough to handle, 5 to 10 minutes.

Holding a corn cob over a large bowl, use a knife to carefully slice warm kernels directly into the bowl; discard cob. Repeat with remaining corn.

Add bell pepper, tomatoes, onion, cilantro, olive oil, salt, and pepper; toss until evenly mixed. Let sit until flavors have blended, at least 30 minutes.

Jicama Mango Salad with Cilantro and Lime

Things To Get

1 large jicama, peeled and cut into matchsticks

1 small red bell pepper, cut into matchsticks

1 large firm mango, peeled and cut into matchsticks

½ red onion, cut into matchsticks

Dressing:

½ cup chopped cilantro leaves

2 limes, juiced

¼ cup honey

1 teaspoon salt

⅛ teaspoon cayenne pepper, or more to taste

Preparation

Toss jicama, red pepper, mango, and red onion together in a large bowl. Set aside.

Stir cilantro, lime juice, honey, salt, and cayenne pepper together in a bowl.

Pour the cilantro mixture over the jicama mixture and toss to coat. Cover the bowl with plastic wrap and refrigerate for at least 15 minutes.

Note:

Make sure that the mango is very firm so that it is easily julienned.

Taco Slaw

Things To Get

½ small head cabbage, chopped

1 carrot, chopped

1 jalapeno pepper, seeded and minced

½ red onion, minced

1 tablespoon chopped fresh cilantro

1 lime, juiced

Preparation

Mix together cabbage, carrot, jalapeño pepper, red onion, cilantro, and lime juice in a bowl.

Very Easy Fruit Salad

Things To Get

1 pint strawberries - cleaned, hulled and sliced

1 pound seedless grapes, halved

3 kiwis, peeled and sliced

3 bananas, sliced

1 (21 ounce) can peach pie filling

Preparation

In a large bowl, combine the strawberries, grapes, kiwis, and bananas. Gently mix in peaches. Chill for 1 hour before serving.

Crisp Marinated Cucumbers

Things To Get

½ cup white vinegar

½ cup white sugar

½ teaspoon salt

¼ teaspoon celery seed

2 medium cucumbers, sliced

¼ cup sliced sweet onion

Preparation

Whisk vinegar, sugar, salt, and celery seed together in a large bow. Add cucumbers and onion and stir until well coated.

Cover and refrigerate 8 hours to overnight. Serve cold.

Freezer Slaw

Things To Get

1 large head cabbage, shredded

1 green bell pepper, finely chopped

1 small small onion, finely chopped

2 carrots, shredded

2 cups boiling water

2 teaspoons salt

1 ½ cups white sugar

1 cup water

¾ cup cider vinegar

2 teaspoons celery seed

Preparation

Combine cabbage, green bell pepper, onion, and carrots in a large bowl. Mix boiling water and salt together in a separate bowl and pour over cabbage mixture; set aside for salt to draw out extra water from vegetables, about 1 hour. Drain well.

Mix sugar, 1 cup water, cider vinegar, and celery seed in a saucepan; bring to a boil. Cook and stir until sugar is dissolved, about 1 minute. Remove the saucepan from the heat and cool completely.

Pour cooled sugar-vinegar mixture over drained cabbage mixture in a large bowl and toss until slaw is well mixed. Spoon slaw into resealable plastic bags; squeeze out excess air, seal the bag, and freeze.

Tips

When ready to use, thaw in the refrigerator, drain excess fluid, and add mayonnaise to suit your taste.

Cucumber Sunomono

Things To Get

2 large cucumbers, peeled

⅓ cup rice vinegar

4 teaspoons white sugar

1 teaspoon salt

1 ½ teaspoons minced fresh ginger root

Preparation

Cut cucumbers in half lengthwise and scoop out any large seeds. Slice crosswise into very thin slices.

In a small bowl combine vinegar, sugar, salt and ginger. Mix well. Place cucumbers inside of the bowl, stir so that cucumbers are coated with the mixture. Refrigerate the bowl of cucumbers for at least 1 hour before serving.

Tomato Cucumber Salad

Things To Get

2 tomatoes, chopped

1 cucumber, peeled and diced

1 onion, chopped

1 tablespoon lemon juice

salt to taste

ground black pepper to taste

Preparation

Combine tomatoes, cucumbers, and onions in a salad bowl. Season to taste with salt and black pepper. Sprinkle with lemon juice. Chill.

Mom's Cucumbers

Things To Get

3 large cucumbers

1 teaspoon salt

¼ cup white sugar

⅛cup water

¼ cup distilled white vinegar

½ teaspoon celery seed

¼ cup chopped onion

Preparation

Peel the cucumbers and slice wafer thin. Sprinkle with salt. Let stand 30 minutes, then squeeze cucumbers to release moisture.

In a medium size bowl mix sugar, water, vinegar, celery seed, and onion. Add cucumbers to mixture. Mix well. Refrigerate 1 hour.

Berry Fruit Salad

Things To Get

1 cup fresh strawberries, hulled and quartered lengthwise

1 cup fresh blueberries

1 cup fresh blackberries

1 cup fresh raspberries

1 teaspoon white sugar

Preparation

Mix strawberries, blueberries, blackberries, and raspberries together in a bowl. Sprinkle with sugar.

Curtido (El Salvadoran Cabbage Salad)

Things To Get

½ head green cabbage, cored and shredded

1 carrot, grated

1 quart boiling water

3 green onions, minced

1 cup distilled white vinegar

½ cup water

2 teaspoons dried oregano

Preparation

Combine the cabbage and carrot in a large bowl and pour the boiling water over the mixture. Allow the mixture to steep for 5 minutes; drain well. Return the cabbage and carrots to the bowl. Mix in the green onion, vinegar, 1/2 cup of water, and oregano. Toss until all **Things To Get** are combined. Chill for 20 minutes before serving.

Dandelion Salad

Things To Get

½ pound torn dandelion greens

½ red onion, chopped

2 tomatoes, chopped

½ teaspoon dried basil

salt and pepper to taste

Preparation

In a medium bowl, toss together dandelion greens, red onion, and tomatoes. Season with basil, salt, and pepper.

Ukrainian Salat Vinaigrette (Beet Salad)

Things To Get

1 pound beets

1 pound carrots

1 pound potatoes

2 large dill pickles, diced

1 onion, minced

1 (8 ounce) can peas, drained

2 tablespoons olive oil

½ teaspoon ground black pepper

1 tablespoon chopped fresh parsley (Optional)

½ teaspoon salt

Preparation

Place the beets into a large pot and cover with water. Bring to a boil over high heat, then reduce heat to medium-low, cover, and simmer for about 20 minutes. Add the carrots and potatoes. Boil for another 10 minutes, then cover the pot and leave overnight.

The next day, peel and dice the beets, carrots, and potatoes into small, even pieces. Place the vegetables in a large bowl. Stir in the pickles, onion, peas, olive oil, salt, and pepper. Garnish with parsley before serving.

Conch Salad

Things To Get

1 pound fresh conch

1 ¼ cups lemon juice, divided

1 cup diced tomatoes

½ cup diced onion

½ cup diced green bell pepper

½ cup diced cucumber

¼ teaspoon seasoning blend (such as Badia®
Complete Seasoning®), or to taste

1 pinch seasoned salt, or to taste

2 cups tomato juice

¼ cup lime juice

¼ cup vinegar

1 dash hot sauce, or to taste

Preparation

Tenderize conch with a meat mallet. Dice into bite-sized chunks. Soak conch in 1 cup lemon juice for at least 2 hours, preferably overnight.

Drain off lemon juice and place conch in a bowl. Add tomatoes, onion, green pepper, cucumber, seasoning blend, and seasoned salt; mix thoroughly.

Transfer conch mixture to a container. Add remaining 1/4 cup lemon juice, tomato juice, and lime juice; mix well. Stir in vinegar and hot sauce. Refrigerate until flavors combine, about 1 hour. Serve cold.

CHAPTER SIX

JUST ONE FINAL THING TO ADDRESS BEFORE YOU GO!

Fatty liver disease, as the name suggests, pertains to a medical condition characterized by the accumulation of fat within the liver. This ailment manifests in two primary forms: alcohol-induced, which arises from excessive alcohol consumption, and nonalcoholic, which can develop irrespective of alcohol intake. While alcoholic fatty liver disease impacts approximately 5% of the population in the United States, nonalcoholic fatty liver disease (NAFLD) poses a more widespread concern, affecting an estimated 100 million individuals in the country. Alarmingly, NAFLD has emerged as the predominant liver disorder among children in the nation.

Nonalcoholic fatty liver steatohepatitis (NASH) represents a more severe variant of NAFLD, marked by inflammation and liver cell damage, potentially progressing to grave complications such as cirrhosis and liver cancer. Addressing the liver's condition, regardless of its etiology, necessitates comprehensive lifestyle modifications. Effective interventions encompass weight loss strategies, abstinence from alcohol consumption, and adherence to a specialized diet tailored to alleviate the burden on the liver.

Understanding the multifaceted nature of fatty liver disease is paramount for implementing targeted interventions and mitigating its detrimental consequences. By fostering awareness and promoting proactive measures, healthcare practitioners and individuals alike can collaboratively combat the pervasive threat of liver disorders.